T0331275

Adult Day Care:
A Practical Guidebook
and Manual

ABOUT THE AUTHORS

Dr. Lenore A. Tate is the Principal Consultant for Mental Health and Developmental Disabilities for the California Assembly. Previously, she has been an Assistant Professor of Adult Development and Aging at Arizona State University and has Chaired the Psychology Program at Prairie View A & M University in Texas. Prior to beginning her professional career, she was selected as a two-year National Institute of Mental Health Post-Doctoral Fellow in Geriatric Psychology by the Texas Research Institute of Mental Sciences in Houston. She obtained her PhD from the California School of Professional Psychology in 1980. She holds an MS from Howard University and a BA from Mills College in Oakland, California.

Dr. Tate has published several articles in gerontology and has held leadership positions in the geriatric community. She has served as a lecturer in several community colleges and in the California State University System. She has presented a numerous gerontological conferences and conventions on a local, national, and international level. As a consultant, Dr. Tate has worked with private industry, universities, and government entities.

Dr. Tate has received numerous awards and recognition for her service to her community. She has been selected as an Outstanding Young Woman of America in 1984. She is also a member of various professional organizations and active in community activities including past board member of the American Society of Aging and an active member of Alpha Kappa Alpha Sorority. She has also lived and studied in Europe and traveled to Northern Africa and the Caribbean.

Cynthia M. Brennan, co-author is currently working for the Area Agency on Aging, Region I and teaches part-time at Mesa Community College in Arizona. Between 1978-1985, she worked for the Foundation for Senior Living both as a program director and later as a field director with responsibilities for nine adult day care centers. Ms. Brennan wishes to acknowledge the Foundation for Senior Living as being a leader in the provision of adult day care services. Ms. Brennan was the first President of the Arizona Association of Adult Day Health Care and has previously served as Region IX representative on the steering committee of the National Institute of Adult Day Care with NCOA. Ms. Brennan holds a Bachelors degree in Sociology and a Masters degree in Public Administration.

Adult Day Care:
A Practical Guidebook and Manual

Lenore A. Tate
Cynthia M. Brennan

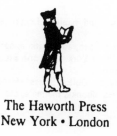

The Haworth Press
New York • London

0-86656-711-9

Adult Day Care: A Practical Guidebook and Manual has also been published as *Activities, Adaptation & Aging*, Volume 11, Number 2 1988.

The Haworth Press, Inc., 10 Alice Street, Binghamton, New York 13904-1580
EUROSPAN/Haworth, 3 Henrietta Street, London, WC2E 8LU England

Library of Congress Cataloging-in-Publication Data

Tate, Lenore A.
Adult day care : a practical guidebook and manual / Lenore A. Tate, Cynthia M. Brennan.
  p. cm.
  "Has also been published as Activities, adaptation & aging, volume 11, number 2, 1988."
  Reprint. Originally published: New York : Haworth Press, ©1988.
  Includes bibliographical references.
  1. Day care centers for the aged—United States—Handbooks, manuals, etc. 2. Aged—Institutional care—United States—Handbooks, manuals, etc. I. Brennan, Cynthia M. II Title.
HV1455.2.U6T37   1990
362.6'3—dc20   89-24498
                                                                                CIP

Dedicated to

My deceased grandparents,
Otto Artie and Emma Ruth Hopkins
and
Mrs. Clara B. Emmett

Adult Day Care:
A Practical Guidebook
and Manual

CONTENTS

Introduction

Since the early 1970s, adult day care centers in the United States have grown from 20 to over 620 centers. Similarly, in Arizona, the Foundation for Senior Living, a nonprofit organization has provided adult day care services to frail and impaired elderly individuals. From three centers in the early 1970s, the Foundation for Senior Living has developed a network of nine adult day care centers that serve urban and rural communities. This rapid increase in adult day care programs suggests that this is an important health care and social resource that has begun to fill a necessary gap in the long-term care system (Pritzlaff Commission, 1984).

The Foundation for Senior Living and other organizations have recognized the need for continuity in long-term care services. Long-term care services include but are not limited to home care, meals-on-wheels, congregate meal centers, senior centers, social and recreational programs, and adult day care. These services represent a new approach in community support systems for the elderly.

As the number of elderly persons increase, demographic trends suggest that the size of the American family will decrease. It is becoming more difficult for small families to provide full-time care for a frail or impaired elderly relative, loved one, or neighbor. Additionally, various social (e.g., work, marriage, retirement, leisure time) or psychological (e.g., stress, depression, late-life expectations) factors also influence the type and quality of caregiving and affect the intermittent level of health care and social services necessary to maintain elderly individuals within their community.

The development of noninstitutionalized community care has become an effective social/health delivery system. While keeping

For reprint requests write to Dr. Lenore A. Tate, Assembly Committee on Health, State Capital, P. O. Box 942849, Sacramento, CA 94249-0001.

1

costs at a minimum (for four million elderly individuals who are severely limited by at least one chronic illness and another four and a half million that have some restricted activity) adult day care centers have provided a supervised and supportive environment for many families.

This guidebook and manual is intended for long-term care providers, consumers, and gerontology students. It provides information regarding (1) the history, definition and concept of adult day care; (2) models of care; (3) scope of activities; (4) state and national policy; and (4) a manual with forms and reports necessary for daily operations. We encourage you to share this monograph with others in order to promote and enhance adult day care as an essential link in long-term care.

Chapter One

·Aging:
A National Perspective

America is a nation that is aging. Elderly persons now comprise the fastest growing segment of the population (Dolan, 1980). Since the baby boom of the 1940s and 1950s, the nation has shifted from a youth-oriented society to an adult-oriented culture. Today, 12.2% of the population is over the age of 65. The increase in the over 65 segment of the population is expected to continue well into the year 2035, when the elderly will comprise 18% of the total population. Within the elderly population, the fastest rate of growth is the "old-old." In this age group, over 10 million persons are over 75 years of age. The number of people aged 85 and over has tripled between 1950 and 1970, increasing from 600,000 to 2 million. The number in the 75 to 85 age group has almost doubled. These are the ages in which hospitalization, institutionalization, and an array of long-term care services are very high (Farber, 1983).

Prior to 1950 many of today's medical procedures were not available, hence many older persons suffered dependency or death. Improvements in sanitation, public health, disease control, medical care, and general quality of life have enhanced the number and proportion of older people in the general population. At the same time many older persons have one or more chronic conditions such as diabetes, cardiovascular disease, arthritis, and impaired vision and hearing (Butler & Lewis, 1982; Golightly et al., 1984). In addition, they are at risk for further decrements and acute exacerbation of their chronic conditions (Brody, 1980). It is not surprising that the average health care usage and cost for older Americans is disproportionately higher than for those persons under the age of 65

3

(Butler & Lewis, 1982; Roos, Shapiro & Roos, 1984; Vital Health Statistics, 1980). The maintenance of adequate health care, then, becomes increasingly more significant to the elderly as they continue to grow older, become more frail, and find their financial resources are limited by a fixed income.

During recent decades, recognizable advances in the health care industry and apparent successes in refinements of care have increased demands for service. National policy reflects a need for affordable and improved care that can be subsidized in one form or another. Programs instituted for older citizens are a result of this policy. Medicare and Medicaid programs that began in the 1960s are now an integral part of United States governmental programs. Today, a variety of proposals are before congressional committees to expand these programs and to add modalities for federal participation.

By the latter part of the 1970s and into the 1980s, a number of states instituted legislation to place limitations on federal government spending. Many social and health programs that grew out of early federal support systems are now obliged to find new alternative funding because of diminishing resources. The rigidity of federal and state reimbursement systems has discouraged the development of activities (McCuan, 1973). Although long-term effects of these changes are not known, many programs have been curtailed. On the other hand, the potential of private insurance (third-party reimbursement) or pension plans are being investigated by many programs.

Quite obviously, the reimbursement source influences the nature of programs and services to the elderly. In view of these convergent and growing needs for innovative approaches to treatment/care for the elderly, a relatively new concept has found its place among the long-term care services. Adult day care is a relatively low-cost service that assists the frail elderly and physically impaired adult by providing personal care, supervision, and an organized program of activities, experiences, and therapies in a protective setting. It offers an individualized plan of care designed to maintain impaired persons at, or restore them to, their optimal level of independence (Padula, 1983). Padula reported that a variety of adult day care programs offer services ranging from active rehabilitation to social and health-related care. These programs are usually coordinated with and related to other agencies and services such as senior centers, in-home care, and institutional and hospital care. Padula concludes that it is an innovative way to organize and blend traditional health and social services for the frail adult.

Adult day care offers several advantages and is distinguished from other forms of long-term care primarily in that " . . . it allows the participant: (1) to continue to live in the home; (2) to maintain social ties in their community; (3) to relieve the family of the burden for 24-hour care; and (4) to be cost-effective" (O'Brien, 1980).

AGING IN ARIZONA

As a result of the increased numbers of elderly and their need for services, Arizona communities began implementing adult day care programs in the 1970s.

Even though tens of thousands of retirees make Arizona their Winter home, the year-round proportion of people 65 and over has been about the same as the national average. Currently, nearly one out of five (20%) Arizona residents are 55 years of age. Eleven percent—more than 307,000 persons—are over the age of 65 in Arizona (see Table 1). The number of elderly people between the ages of 75 to 85 years is increasing rapidly. This age group comprises 38% of the elderly and will rise to 44% in the next 16 years. While the elderly share common problems, persons 75 years of age and older are the most vulnerable to physical, mental, and social problems that lead to requests for health care and related services.

Approximately 80% of all persons over the age of 65 have at least one chronic disease, 30 to 40% of those over 65 have significant hearing or visual impairments, and 25 to 30% of those over 65 have some evidence of dementia or depression. As these statistics indicate, the state of Arizona, and Phoenix in particular, is in urgent need of a coordinated care program. An effective program consists of a balance of appropriate social and supportive services; acute and long-term care (skilled, intermediate, and supervisory); and innovative, preventive, diagnostic, and rehabilitative services (e.g., adult day care, home health care, nutrition, live-in care, social activity, and hospice).

Table 1.   1980 Census Population 65 Years and Over.

	United States	Arizona
White	22,948,193	285,664
Black	2,086,858	5,087
Native American, Eskimos, and Aleut	74,919	7,135
Asian/Pacific Islander	211,736	1,084
Other	227,721	8,393
Total population 65+	25,549,427	307,362
Spanish Origin*	708,880*	19,797*

*May be any race.

Source: U.S. Department of Commerce, Bureau of the Census. (1983).

The providers of long-term care, acute care, and supportive, rehabilitative, and social care in Arizona are involved in developing networks and health care delivery systems to increase their share of the elderly market and related reimbursable health care services. The state of Arizona and leading employers (Arizona Coalition for Cost-Effective Quality Health Care) as well as health care insurers are stressing the importance of cost containment and/or responsible and efficient management by health care resources.

Currently, there is no licensing of adult day care in the state of Arizona. Programs which receive federal dollars go through a certification process authorized by the Department of Economic Security. The Arizona Association of Adult Day Health Care is supportive of "some kind" of licensing requirements and standards for adult day care centers in Arizona. A study committee formed by the Department of Health Services (DHS) has submitted a draft of proposed recommendations for the licensing of adult day care/adult day health care to the Director of DHS. This committee was represented by people throughout the state who had knowledge of adult day care and who worked for 10 months on these recommendations.

In Arizona, families of the elderly and disabled provide approximately 80% of the support services necessary to maintain the elderly in their communities. Various studies indicate that families today are smaller, and often both husband and wife are employed away from home. Care for the elderly at home becomes increasingly difficult without proper community support and resources.

In Arizona, most community programs for the elderly are provided by nonprofit groups such as the Foundation for Senior Living (FSL), incorporated in 1974. FSL's founders believed that support and advocacy services for older Americans should be provided to meet the steady increase of elderly in the population. FSL provides a complete range of programs, services, and facilities to meet the varied needs of older Americans. These include community service activities, live-in care, nutrition programs, Retired Senior Volunteer Program (RSVP), retirement housing, nursing homes, homemaker services, home health care, and adult day care. FSL has over 8,500 senior participants in five counties within the state of Arizona: Maricopa, Mohave, Yavapai, Yuma, and Coconino. It employs approximately 400 persons on a full- or part-time basis to administer, staff, and provide a wide range of health and community services to the elderly of Arizona. A professional staff manages FSL under the guidance of a volunteer board of directors consisting of 30 members who are elected on an annual basis.

A portion of FSL's funding comes from federal, state, and local government grants. Agencies providing funding for FSL's programs include the Area Agency on Aging, Department of Economic Security, Maricopa County Human Resources, Department of Action, and City of Phoenix. The balance of the funding is received from contributions, private grants, United Way, corporate gifts, individual fees, rental income, and management fees.

Adult day care centers were one of the Foundation for Senior Living's original programs and FSL has gained respect from the community for its effort in preventing premature or inappropriate institutionalization. FSL's adult day care programs are among the finest in the country and have been so mentioned in national publications (Leonard, 1978). Despite recent funding reductions, the

Foundation opened four new adult day care programs in areas of need, and continued to provide the highest quality of adult day care services.

HISTORY

Adult day care was initially associated with psychiatric patients and began in the U.S.S.R. in 1942. By 1946, day care facilities opened in London and Montreal. In the United States, the Menninger Clinic and the Yale Psychiatric Clinic opened on an experimental basis (Dolan, 1980). However, it was not until 1958 that the first geriatric day hospital was built at the United Oxford Hospital in London (Cosin et al., 1958). This acute-care program was designed to return the elderly person back home. It included a thorough diagnostic examination and an individual treatment plan which stressed activities which included daily living skills and supportive community involvement (e.g., homemaker services, ambulance service, physical and occupational therapy, senior centers, etc.). Geriatric day care is now considered an integral part of geriatric care in England (Padula, 1983).

The adult day care movement in this country began in 1958 with a three-year project in a day hospital rehabilitative program in Schenectady, New York. By 1969, a subcommittee of the Maryland Department of Health and Mental Hygiene issued its findings about the purpose and requirements of day care for the elderly (Padula, 1983). Adult day care centers then began to develop throughout the nation.

Tucson's Senior Health Improvement Program was one of the first adult day care programs started in the United States in 1972. FSL began planning for adult day care in 1972 and opened its first adult day care center in 1973. Since 1973 it has increased to nine centers. FSL operates more adult day care facilities than any other organization in the state of Arizona. Currently seven of the nine centers in Arizona are operating at full capacity (20-40 clients per day depending on the physical size of the building) Monday through Friday.

The number of adult day care centers has increased in the United

States from 12 programs in the 1960s to 20 in the 1970s to over 1,200 in the 1980s. These centers serve over 18,000 persons daily.

Models of Adult Day Care

Adult day care has been applied to a spectrum of uniquely different services designed for elderly persons with varying levels of need. No one model of adult day care can serve all who need such services but it is possible that in some instances a specific program can serve two or more levels of care. Most adult day care centers describe their program by utilizing one of three types of program models. Currently these models include (1) the *health* or *restorative* model which in some states is Medicaid reimbursable (28 states reimburse for adult day care),[1] (2) the *maintenance* model, and (3) the *(psycho) social* model which is often supported by Title XX funds. Each of the three models have commonalities such as psychosocial activities to improve and maintain mental health, health supervision and supportive services, nutrition services including noonday meals and snacks, and transportation (see Table 2).

Model I. The health or restorative model emphasizes medical and/or rehabilitation services along with health supportive services for participants who might otherwise be placed in a skilled nursing home if this form of care were not available. The participant is expected to improve within the confines of a limited time span. Any needed supplemental home health services may be provided by public health nurses, home health aides, or physical or speech therapists.

The participants receive one-to-one therapeutic services from certified specialists. Physicians are not a part of this model; continuing medical care is the responsibility of each participant's personal physician. The personal physician makes recommendations for care that will be incorporated into the care plan by the center's multidisciplinary team.

Model II. The maintenance model is a combination of the restorative and social models. It usually provides long-term maintenance services to a high-risk population who either are eligible for institutional care or could reasonably be expected to be eligible for such care in the near future if continuous health monitoring and support-

Table 2.   Three Models of Adult Day Care*

MODEL	CLIENTS	SERVICES OFFERED	DAYS/ WEEK OFFERED	ESTI- MATED COST	EXPECTED OUTCOME	FAMILY RESPONSIBILITY	COMMUNITY SUPPORTS
Health or restor- ative	Severely disabled, post- hospital post- nursing home	Intensive restorative medical and health serv- ices (P.T., O.T., S.T.), activities, nutrition	5 Days	$20- 30/ day	Higher level of function- ing both physical and mental	Training of family members to give care on weekends and nights	Usually are necessary
Main- tenance	"At-risk" popula- tion	Long-term health maintenance services, nursing services, activities, nutrition	5 Days	$10- 25/ day	Preven- tion of institu- tionali- zation, relief to families, promotion of health	Families provide health super- vision in home during days not at program	Offered when necessary
Psycho- social	Socially isolated, "frail elderly," slightly disabled	Psychosocial Activities in a protect- ed environ- ment, nutri- tion	5 Days	$5- 15/ day	Prevent mental deterior- ation and physical breakdown, promotion of health	Families provide supervision at home if necessary	Not usually necessary

*Adapted from the four models of adult day care by Edith Robins in "Operational Research in
.Geriatric Day Care in the United State," paper presented at the 105th International Gerontological Congress, Jerusalem, Israel, June, 1985.

ive services were not provided. The participants are provided with supervised activities, psychosocial services, and health monitoring. This type of program is recommended by a physician or a patient is referred by a clinic, and a treatment plan is developed by the adult day care center's multidisciplinary team. This type of care often provides essential physical relief to caregivers in their efforts to maintain the individual in the home, or it provides essential supervision during the hours when family members are at work and there is no one in the home to give the needed care and/or supervision. FSL offers long-term maintenance programs for the frail elderly and chronically disabled adult.

Model III. The (psycho) social model is varied and there is no typical program. Services emphasize socialization and range from lunches to geriatric linkages in the community to nursing services and health care maintenance services. Usually this model attempts to prevent or decelerate mental and/or physical deterioration. Activities are encouraged and attendance is on a regular basis. Professional staff usually include a social worker (preferably with gerontology training), a part-time nurse, activity coordinator, geriatric aides, and volunteers. Clients of FSL's psychosocial adult day care program receive an individualized program of care and are monitored within a group setting. The many services provided within FSL operated programs include nutrition, transportation, structured activities (e.g., arts, crafts, drama, music, etc.), physical and speech therapy, reality orientation, psychosocial therapies, and exercises.

PARTICIPANTS

Since Arizona is composed of many different ethnic groups it is suggested that their cultural values be respected in planning and operating a day care program. For example, the center should take into account food preferences, special holidays, minority/majority cultural values, bilingual staff, gender roles, and attitudes towards persons in authority.

A "micro" perspective of the diagnostic typology of day care participants is varied. Most adult day care participants are either disabled, depressed, or disoriented to the degree that they cannot function as independent adults. Loss (due to status, responsibilities, significant others, or health) is a predominant theme with the elderly and may result in depression. Other psychological problems and inappropriate behaviors include suspiciousness, paranoid ideations, incontinence, agitation, wandering, loss of interest, and grief. Thus with the aging experience may come feelings and behaviors that reflect life events of this population. Some participants live alone and cannot totally care for themselves. Others live with families and adult day care relieves the family of total responsibility so that the participant can continue to live at home while their adult children may work or have some respite. Individuals who are discharged from an institutional setting and need support in order to return to normal activities within their community are encouraged to participate in FSL's adult day care.

FSL adult day care centers will not admit an individual who is bedridden, a substance abuser, is harmful to him/herself or to others, does not have medical need, or is unwilling to attend. A perusal of the centers shows that there are approximately eight incontinent participants per center.

The "typical" profile of a FSL participant is a Caucasian widowed female who is approximately 77.5 years old and living with her family. She usually has 10 to 12 years of education, an income ceiling of $499 per month, and is funded for day care by Title XX. She is oriented, can walk a maximum of one city block, and has had a stroke and/or mental health-related disorder.

Adult day care provides a safe and stimulating environment for the frail and/or disabled adult while other family members are at work. Its services try to assist the demented in maintaining daily living skills. Further adult day care provides psychosocial stimulation, socialization, and nutrition in a protective environment.

FSL's current programs assist the elderly by restoring or maintaining their capacity to be active in their community. The participant learns to adapt to the physical world and gradually resumes the normal activities required in daily living. The participant is taught to fully use his/her intellectual, social, and physical potentials. For the older participant, activities of daily living become a primary area of focus.

FSL and adult day care staff try to promote a "caring" attitude toward each participant. The word "care" as used by FSL is derived from the Latin word "caritas," meaning respect, esteem, affection, and value. FSL's staff represent a shift in thinking that the frail person has little or no value; instead, the staff's attitude of "caring" focuses on concern for the well-being and social integration of the participant. Therefore, the services, programs, and treatment plans generally require innovative and careful planning.

SERVICES

The service program defines the population served, the purpose(s) of the adult day care center, and the individual service needs of the participant group. When any services introduced address an identified need, the center has a greater chance to succeed. Adaptation in services provided may be modified or changed over time depending on the participant's status.

Core services essential in any adult day care setting include transportation, health surveillance, a hot noon meal, counseling, activities, exercise, and rest. All services need to take place in a safe and stimulating environment. Additional services offered by many adult day care programs include special diets; personal care services; physical, occupational, and speech therapy; training in the use of environmental aids; evaluation of the home setting with suggestions for easing tasks of daily living; individual and group counseling for families and caregivers of the frail elderly; nutrition and consumer education; and self-care health skills; skilled nursing and medical specialists; and a variety of peripheral services like shopping, laundry, barber and beauty shops, etc.

Generally, FSL's adult day care centers include the following services:

1. Nutritional services—which include one noon meal, two snacks, and nutritional counseling.
2. Health services—reliable health supervision and health counseling are available, usually from a registered nurse.
3. Recreational and social activities—planned for the levels of need of each participant.
4. Information and referral services—provide information regarding social, psychological, and medical services with referrals to agencies, clinics, and medical specialists as needed or requested.
5. Social services—provide assessment, counseling, and long-term care planning.
6. Van transportation to and from the center.
7. Student internships—provided in law, social work, psychology, nursing, art, and recreation.

8. Therapies such as physical, speech, and occupational are provided at each center by contracting with rehabilitation agencies.

FAMILY INVOLVEMENT AND RESPONSIBILITY

Family members are encouraged to become involved in FSL's adult day care program. The family, the client, and the staff try to work together to understand the needs of the participant. Strategies are developed which will best meet the participant's needs at home and at the center to provide 24-hour continuity of care. All staff are prepared to help families or to make appropriate referrals.

Family members must leave emergency telephone numbers in the event the participant requires immediate attention. If necessary, the staff or paramedics will transport a client to the nearest medical emergency room.

Part of FSL's philosophy assumes that within reasonable limits the potential participant has the right to make decisions for him/herself, with the help of significant family members, about his/her life. FSL asserts that this decision-making process helps to maintain and/or improve an individual's self-esteem and intellectual functioning.

Many of FSL's adult day care participants have been with the program since 1973. A family-like atmosphere coupled with an interest and concern by the staff have provided support to both the participant and his/her family in these centers. Frequently during a family crisis, the adult day care director has been known to provide emotional support, informational and referral service, and assistance to the family of the client. Most staff and participants choose to attend the funeral services when a member of the adult day care center dies.

PERSONNEL

Staff needs vary in each FSL adult day care center, depending on the various demographic characteristics and the services offered. In FSL-operated adult day care centers, staff include a full-time director, an activity coordinator, a social worker, a registered nurse, and a van driver. There may also be geriatric aides, student interns, a secretary, and volunteers from within the community.

FSL's staff consist of a carefully selected and trained group of individuals who are able to cope with behaviors generally viewed as "inappropriate" or "threatening" to others. These behaviors include confusion and disorientation which are occasionally followed by hygienic accidents and verbal abuse or combative behaviors. Even with the high-demand, high-stressed environment, staff turnover is low. For example, the highest staff turnover occurs with activity coordinators and social workers who remain with the program for approximately 12 months. The adult day care directors remain with the center at least four years while most of the remaining staff (nurses, group directors, aides, clerical, and drivers) have been with the program since 1973 (FSL files, 1985).

Staffing

FSL's staff-to-participant ratio is higher than the minimum requirements set by Arizona's Department of Economic Security to provide quality care and adequate supervision. The state of Arizona requires two staff for up to 10 patients, three for 11 to 20 clients, four for 21 to 30 clients, and five for 31 to 40 clients. FSL usually has two staff for every 10 clients, four for 11 to 20 clients, six for 21 to 30 clients, and eight for 31 to 40 clients, along with volunteers for additional help with supervision.

A staff ratio of one staff person for each eight clients, excluding the director, is the suggested guideline nationally (National Institute of Adult Day-Care, 1984). In Arizona, for those programs receiving federal funding, the minimum requirements match the national standards (Department of Economic Security, 1977). Realistically, the director of the program should not be counted as part of the staff requirements because much of his/her time will be spent in administering or evaluating the program, developing community support, consulting with other agencies and organizations, meeting with the advisory board, recruiting and supervising staff, and in preparing reports. Volunteers are valuable adjuncts to assist with supervision and should not be considered as paid staff in the above ratios.

Programs throughout the country have varying staff compositions according to the *Directory of Adult Day Care Centers* published by the Health Care Financing Administration in 1980. A few adult day care centers have entirely volunteer staffs, some share staff with other programs (nursing homes and/or senior centers), and one mental health program has 22 staff members for a program that serves 40 people per day.

A typical staffing pattern follows:

1. *Director, full-time*
2. *Social Worker(s)*
   a. Serves as assistant director when director is away.
   b. Handles individual and group counseling, casework, and accession services.
   c. In adult day care, the social worker is closely involved with each participant and his/her family or caregiver. The social work services may include:
      — Assisting a client to get new eyeglasses.
      — Riding with the client to the hospital in the ambulance when an emergency occurs.
      — Choosing to attend funerals.
      — Assisting families with funeral arrangements as it becomes necessary.
3. *Activity Coordinator and Activity Aides*
   The activity coordinator and aides are needed to carry out concurrent activities and to provide assistance with physical exercise, educational programs, and productive activities.
4. *Registered Nurse*
   A registered nurse is needed — at least on a part-time basis — to provide health surveillance for clients.
5. *Secretary*
   A secretary is needed to answer the telephone, type reports, maintain records/files, fill out monthly reports, bill clients, and serve as a receptionist.
6. *Bookkeeper*
   Bookkeeping services are needed to set up and maintain purchasing records, monitor ledgers, accounts payable, accounts receivable, and assure periodic audits of the accounts. A board member or volunteer from the community may assist with some of these tasks.

7. *Van Driver(s)*

If an adult day care center has its own van, one or more drivers will be needed. Driver alertness is enhanced when two part-time drivers are used, one for the morning shift and one for the afternoon shift.

8. *Janitor(s)/Custodian(s)*

Janitorial services are usually provided on a contractual basis.

9. *Cook*

Most adult day care centers cater their food, but a cook is needed if the meals are prepared on-site.

The secretary, driver(s), and cook positions should not be counted as part of the staff ratio except for the time they may provide direct service to the participants.

There are special qualities an individual staff member must have to successfully work with geriatric participants: patience, a cheerful disposition, a genuine "liking" for older people, honesty, dependability, cooperativeness, adaptability, sincerity, unselfishness, good manners, tact, and competence. Moreover, while working with the participants the staff should try to view the interrelationship between body, mind, and environment since change in one of these may cause change in another.

Written job descriptions and definition of responsibility help each person see how his/her position fits into the overall adult day care operation (Appendix L). Job descriptions work as a guide but must convey flexibility when the need arises. Job specifications for the director establishing lines of authority for hiring and firing, expenditures and budget preparation, policy changes, etc., should be clearly stated.

No matter how an adult day care center is staffed, volunteers play a conspicuous role in all adult day care programs. Volunteers are a particularly important link in enhancing the quality of adult day care for the participant. Their skills enrich the program. Assignments given to volunteers in the adult day care programs may be chosen from the following areas: (1) administrative or advisory help, (2) group leadership, (3) nonleadership roles, (4) clerical or maintenance work, and (5) miscellaneous services. Specific activities in which volunteers could assist include: (1) leading special groups such as current events, travel, reminiscing, writing, and gardening;

(2) assisting the activity coordinator in the arts and crafts program; (3) assisting in reality orientation groups; and (4) accompanying participants to special outings and events such as dances, dinners, and parties.

Another important role for volunteers in adult day care activity programs is that of providing entertainment for the residents. It is important that potential entertainment be screened and any necessary adaptations made to ensure the presentation is appropriate. Volunteers are among the best supporters of a program. In addition to helping within a center, they spread the word about adult day care to potential clients and funding sources and evoke public interest. Volunteers should have orientation sessions and know clearly who is responsible for their activities and to whom they may address their questions (see Appendix I for FSL's Volunteer Policies).

Working together as a team in the interest of participants is not always easy. Freedom and discipline are both required. Philosophies and objectives need to be clear, allowing for maximum inventiveness to carry them out. Everyone needs to be appreciated, especially among the staff. Staff meetings on a weekly basis serve to pull together the various components of adult day care.Staff members with less formal education and gerontological interns may need encouragement to speak up, but their perspective is often valuable and intuitive.

IN-SERVICE TRAINING

Pioneering the way for quality personnel within FSL's organization, a systematic in-service training program for all staff is provided by qualified gerontologists. For example, at FSL a geropsychologist directed a three-part training series in normal aging, abnormal aging, and special topics in aging. The gerontology in-service training program was designed to help improve the quality of adult day care services by enhancing the knowledge, skills, and leadership of staff and volunteers (full- and part-time). The general purpose of the training program was two-fold: It increased the awareness of the aging process and presented practical approaches to problems through lectures, discussions, and role playing.

Numerous studies have been conducted on the topic of curriculum development and in-service training in the field of gerontology (Ernst & Shore, 1977; Hickey, 1974; Spear, 1970). Effective training ensures an adequate supply of staff who are knowledgeable about the aging process and sensitive to the varied social and cultural patterns of the elderly. The Gerontological Society of America, the Association for Gerontology in Higher Education, and the President's 1979 Commission on Mental Health have recommended that in-service training be provided for current staff and related personnel who serve the elderly.

Training probably should be presented in both didactic and experiential modes. The format should be flexible so that the trainer can modify each session according to the specific needs of the staff and their participants. The FSL training program consisted of three general content areas: biological, psychological, and social aspects of aging. Generally, the training attempted to: (1) increase basic understanding of aging principles; (2) provide some structure, content, and process of doing group work with the frail/impaired elderly; and (3) increase understanding of ethnic/minority elders.

Generally, the training sessions attempted to summarize some of the developments and facts affecting the elderly. Table 3 provides a very brief description of the program.

While the above in-service training was valuable and necessary to improve the quality of staff and volunteers, it did not ensure the same quality of service to older minority participants. Thus, the ethnic/minority aging session was included in the in-service training program. It was designed to teach staff how to modify their traditional approaches and to begin to develop culturally responsive interventions, strategies, and approaches. This program was aimed at four ethnic/minority elderly groups: Black (Afro-Americans, West Indians, and others of African descent); Hispanics (Mexican-Americans, Cubans, Puerto Ricans, El Salvadorans, Argentinians, Central and South Americans); Native Americans (all American Indian tribes and Eskimos); and Asians (Koreans, Japanese, Filipinos, Chinese, Vietnamese, and Samoans).

The ethnic/minority aging session covered various cultural differences and similarities that may affect the treatment given to an older ethnic/minority day care participant. It explored cultural life-styles and customs; the status of ethnic/minority older persons; health

Table 3.   In-Service Training in Gerontology

I.   Overview

   A.   History of gerontology

   B.   Palmore's Facts on Aging Quiz (Palmore, 1977)

   C.   Myths vs. facts and realities of aging

   D.   Normal development vs. abnormal age changes

      1.   Common diseases in late life

      2.   Life expectancies/survival rates

II.   Health Issues

   A.   Chronic illnesses

   B.   Pharmacological issues

      1.   Compliance/noncompliance

      2.   Drug interactions and usage

III.   Psychological aspects of aging

   A.   Personality development in late life

   B.   Learning and memory

   C.   Sensory and psychomotor changes with age

   D.   Chronic vs. acute brain syndrome

   E.   Functional disorders

   F.   Sexuality

IV.   Social aspects of aging

   A.   Informal vs. formal support systems

   B.   Death, dying and bereavement

   C.   Recognizing and dealing with "burnout"

   D.   Ethnicity/minority aging

concerns; and the relationship between the family, the community, and other social networks utilized by the four ethnic groups (see Table 4).

It was hoped that a cross-cultural perspective would emerge

Table 4. Ethnicity and Aging.
Purpose

> To inform participants of the general profile of America's older ethnic minority groups. Successful training would facilitate in a better understanding and greater sensitivity toward ethnic minority older persons by increasing their awareness of cultural circumstances. In doing so, the staff will begin to integrate and modify their approaches to effectively serve the day care participant.

Overview

> Training provides information on four ethnic minority groups: Asians, Blacks, Hispanics, and Native Americans. It also provided suggestions of alternatives/strategies for working with minority elders.

Training Outline

I. Introduction

     A. Attitudes and knowledge about minority aging

     B. Personal anxieties

II. Overview of the four ethnic minority groups

     A. The status of the Asian elder

        1. Demographics and epidemiological information

        2. Brief history

        3. Cultural variations

           a. Language

           b. Diet

           c. Religion, activities, and leisure

           d. Strengths

     B. The status of the Black elder

        1. Demographics and epidemiological information

        2. Brief history

        3. Cultural variations

           a. Language

           b. Diet

Table 4 (continued)

    c. Religion, activities, and leisure

    d. Strengths

C. The status of the Hispanic elder

    1. Demographics and epidemiological information

    2. Brief history

    3. Cultural variations

        a. Language

        b. Diet

        c. Religion, activities, and leisure

        d. Strengths

D. The status of the Native American elder

    1. Demographics (number of tribes)

    2. Brief history

    3. Cultural variations

        a. Language

        b. Diet

        c. Religion, activities, and leisure

        d. Strengths

which would help staff understand and appreciate how others live. The overall in-service training session was beneficial to staff who had never had any gerontological training and also for those who may have some experiential background with the elderly but who have not been able to integrate those experiences into their intervention(s) and/or approaches.

TRANSPORTATION

Transportation to and from the adult day care center is essential for the program to operate. Van transportation is usually available and covers target areas usually defined for each center. One of the primary considerations in planning the van route is that no participant rides the van any longer than 30 to 45 minutes. Vans are equipped with lifts and can accommodate wheelchairs.

The van drivers are trained in cardiopulmonary resuscitation (CPR) and first aid. They are trained to be good observers as to changes in the participant's behavior and his/her home environment. Typically FSL's van drivers honk twice and knock at the door to indicate to the participant that the adult day care center's van has arrived. Despite the high-risk population, van transportation has had a low accident rate.

Expense

Transportation is expensive. Gas, oil, and general maintenance costs must be considered. Transportation expenditures may be supplemented by limited Title III and Title XX funds. Transportation expense may be partially paid by client fees, donations, and contributions.

Problems

Many adult day care directors have admitted that transportation is a "headache." The innumerable problems include:

1. When the van needs repair, there usually is no back-up van and staff must transport participants.
2. Often the participants are not ready when the van arrives at their home. The driver may need to coax the participant. Thus, a very flexible driver is needed.
3. Transportation systems for older populations frequently cannot adapt to the frail elderly or the additional number of wheelchairs.
4. Funding for transportation is scarce and highly competitive. There is never enough money to cover all transportation costs.

GENERAL OPERATING BUDGET

Most of the adult day care programs operate on a budget based on the average number of participants (a minimum of 20) attending per day. Transportation to and from the center is included in the budget. The formula to determine the client fee per hour is as follows:

1. Participants per day times days of operation times number of hours per day = total hours/units per year.
2. Total budget ÷ total hours/units per year = hourly rate. For example: 20 participants × 252 operating days × six hours per day = 30,240 hours/units per year. Total budget $87,192 ÷ 30,240 hours/units per year = $2.88 per hour.

Sliding fees are available for those participants and their families who do not qualify for government funding but can not afford to pay the entire fee. These scholarship funds are usually raised by the advisory board and director of each adult day care center. Costs per day include:

1. Noon meal and two snacks.
2. Supervision by a registered nurse.
3. Counseling services for participants and their families.
4. Social services for participants and their families.
5. General care and supervision.
6. Activities and supplies.
7. Transportation (depending on the center's funding, there is usually an additional fee).

Funding

Most adult day care centers use a combination of funding sources to support their program. Usually, funding is difficult to acquire and, in the first few years of operation, often tenuous. It is very important not to rely totally on government revenue to fund an adult day care program. When seeking funding sources, one should always keep in mind client fees and donations; United Way agencies (although this may limit other fund-raising activities); developing an auxiliary, private foundations, and grants; and local staff or board of directors for community fund-raising activities.

Funding for adult day care is usually a composite of funds from Social Service Block Grants (Title XX), the Older American Act (Title III), the Department of Labor (Title V), the United Way, scholarship funds, and private donations. In some other states Medicaid waiver is available under Title XIX. Most centers have periodic fund-raising events and sell crafts produced by clients.

Funds are often administered by state agencies responsible for Title XIX state plans (e.g., Department of Human Resources, Department of Health Services, etc.). The federal Health Care Financing Administration (HCFA) offers technical assistance to states interested in providing adult day care under Medicaid (Bourque, 1984; HCFA, 1980).

Recently, HCFA was given new authority to grant Medicaid waivers for some social adult day health services. Arizona, at this time, is the only state that does not have a Medicaid program and, therefore, does not receive any Medicaid waivers to finance adult day care.

Title XX is part of the Social Security amendments of 1974. Most Title XX dollars are directed toward social service programs. There are income criteria that must be met in order to be eligible for services. Funds are administered through state agencies (Department of Social Services, Department of Economic Security, etc.). Title XX funds more than elderly services; they also fund services for the physically/developmentally disabled children and adults. In recent years, Title XX funding has been drastically reduced at the federal level, making these funding dollars scarce.

Title III of the Older Americans Act of 1965 has various categories of funding. Specifically, Title IIIB dollars (Supportive Services and Senior Centers) and Title IIIC (Nutrition Services) have historically been used to fund adult day care. Title III funds may be used for social, recreational, educational, transportational, and nutritional services. Funds are administered by each state through the local area agencies on aging.

Funding for FSL's adult day care centers is derived from Title XX, county revenue sharing, Title IIIB, and United Way. Fees, contributions, and private donations also provide funding for adult day care (see Appendix M for staff salaries and estimated budget).

A minimum of $60,000 is needed to begin an adult day care

program. Start-up funds are required for supplies, furniture, salaries, etc. A one-time grant or fund-raising activity may make this possible. New centers require about 18 months to recruit sufficient clients and operate a program in the black. As a result the support of an umbrella agency, government, United Way funds, or backing from the community is most essential. It is very difficult to operate on an entirely fee-for-service basis.

Since late December of 1981, the Economic Recovery Tax Act has allowed a tax credit to families with elderly dependents who participate in adult day care centers. The Act established a sliding scale that gives the biggest tax break to families earning $10,000 or less a year. (Check with your local government's regulations.)

CHOOSING A SITE

The most favorable adult day care site is one that has been designed specifically for adult day care. However, the site costs can vary widely. At FSL, the buildings for El Rinconcito, Sirrine, and Prescott Adult Day Care Centers were designed specifically for adult day care. If finances are a problem, a church or school facility is a more economical alternative. Three of the benefits of sharing sites with another organization include reduced costs, the building of community relations and visibility, and the providing of a probable pool of volunteers.

The adult day care philosophy has been to provide an alternative to premature institutionalization. A community-based facility separated from a nursing home or hospital enhances the opportunity to provide a "well" model approach (Padula, 1983). Moreover, the population needing care should be challenged and encouraged physically, mentally, and emotionally if community-based living is to continue. Contrary to the FSL approach, the trend in many nursing homes is to provide adult day care services as a good marketing approach to increase profits or at least as a vehicle to absorb overhead.

This financial incentive may influence nursing homes not to increase the level of a participant's functional independence. The nursing home approach to adult day care services seems to go against the therapeutic philosophy to keep the frail elderly and the disabled as healthy and independent as possible. Moreover, some researchers (Padula, 1983; Snider, 1976) have suggested that a decrease in independent living occurs when attending an adult day care center in a nursing home facility. On the other hand, it may also be noted that nursing home programs may provide evening respite care for families or spouses unlike FSL and other traditionally-based adult day care centers.

PHYSICAL FACILITY

Adult day care is a community-based service located within a community and outside of an institution or nursing home. Adult day care centers may be housed within the building used by the sponsoring organization if space is available. In other instances, adult day care programs are located in space that is rented or obtained free from organizations other than its sponsor—for instance in school buildings, churches, or other municipal buildings.

There are hurdles to overcome regardless of where the adult day care center is located. Rent may be so costly that services must be cut in order to remain within an already tight budget. Many times an adult day care program is sponsored by an already existing organization that may have different goals and objectives than the adult day care program. In this case the adult day care program may have difficulty in maintaining its own goals, staffing pattern, and procedures. If, as in other states, the adult day care program is located within a nursing home or mental institution, there may be difficulty in attracting participants. In addition there may be a crossover of purposes when a nursing home or institution is trying to keep their beds at full capacity. A free-standing adult day care program is usually ideal in that it allows maximum freedom to pursue its own ideas, to enlist cooperation from many sectors of the community, and to have more choice about location.

The physical facility, its location, safety, comfort, and suitability for whatever activities are planned, will either facilitate or complicate the program. Mostly, adult day care programs take what is available, and if fortunate, have the funds needed for essential renovations. There are a few adult day care centers that are very attractive, but for the most part, the participants (or their adult children) make necessary accommodations in order to attend.

The location for the facility should be close to an area where many older people live. Census tract maps and local demographics should all be reviewed before selecting a site because a lack of transportation is one of the major obstacles to servicing seniors.

The average attendance at most adult day care centers is between 20 and 70 people. However, programs with attendance between 30 and 40 seem to be most manageable. The frequency of attendance is determined by the individual need of each participant and is decided upon by the individualized plan of care.

Each state may have minimum requirements or standards having to do with the space required to operate an adult day care program. The amount and variety of space needed will largely depend on the average daily attendance and the kinds of services the center plans to provide. The National Institute of Adult Day Care has just adopted national standards that recommend 40 square feet per person, excluding office, kitchen, or restrooms (NIAD/NCOA, 1984).

The activity room should have as much flexibility as possible to insure the accommodation of changing needs and to allow participants to choose activities for themselves. Secondly, social spaces should be provided where use and desire can be assured (Green, 1975). A good example of this would be a small lounge area in the room in which blood pressures are taken.

The activity room should be large enough to accommodate everyone, including participants, staff, and volunteers at one time. This multipurpose room will be used for large group activities including eating, discussions, and special entertainment. Smaller rooms should be available in order to run concurrent activities such as reality orientation, arts and crafts, range of motion exercises, and any therapies a program might provide. One room should be set aside to allow privacy for interviewing and counseling and an additional room for people who may need to lie down when they are tired or not feeling well. Office space is needed for the director, activity coordinator, social worker, secretary, and files.

Bathrooms must be designed to be wheelchair-accessible and have grab bars in each of the stalls. Older persons use bathroom facilities more frequently and take longer in doing so than do younger people. They must get to the restroom quickly. Consequently, there should be more toilets than are usually required and within easy access. The National Institute of Adult Day Care has adopted standards that include guidelines for bathroom design (NIAD/NCOA, 1984). Green (1975) recommends that each bathroom have sinks that are firmly supported to withstand pulling or leaning loads of up to 300 pounds. The installation should also allow for people using wheelchairs. Instead of round knobs on sinks and doors, levers or cross-shaped knobs should be utilized to allow use by those with coordination and/or dexterity problems.

When possible, there should be a small residential-type kitchen — even if meals are catered — to be used for the retraining of daily living skills, preparation of snacks, and for special holidays or events.

Safety and comfort are prerequisites of all adult day care centers. Crowding is undesirable; people who use walkers, canes, or wheelchairs need free space in order to safely ambulate by themselves. Adult day care centers serve a very fragile population, so the environment should be as barrier-free as possible to keep falls to a minimum.

Listed below are some of the issues one must consider before beginning an adult day care center in any location.

Safety Requirements

1. To comply with local fire and health department regulations, special attention must be given to the number of people who can be safely accommodated in the center's space as well as examining food preparation, serving, and dishwashing safeguards.
2. In case of emergency, there must be at least two exits within easy access of older people whose movements may be slow and unsteady. Additional wheelchairs that may be used for emergencies are essential. Each door must be clearly marked as a fire exit, and each exit must open into an unenclosed outdoor space.
3. Each center must be equipped with a medical kit. Emergency procedures should be posted by each telephone, and telephones must be available to staff at all times.

4. Locked cabinets are a must to store medications.
5. Rooms must be barrier-free, well-lighted, and floors should have a nonslip, level surface to prevent possible falls.

Important Considerations

1. First-floor locations are recommended.
2. Outside ramps should be available.
3. Hand rails installed along inner walls and paths leading to and from the center.
4. Low pile carpeting, if carpeting is used at all. Nonskid flooring is preferable. Coverings should be of one design to prevent distractions when walking.
5. Lever or cross-shaped handles on doors and sinks are easier than round knobs.
6. Grab bars at toilets and urinals, and call lights and/or emergency buzzers should be in each bathroom.
7. Sturdy furniture that will not tip or slide when used for support while walking or sitting down. Chairs with arms are a must for those who have had strokes or who are deemed "unsafe" to sit in a chair without support. Chairs must also be sturdy enough to withstand being moved from place to place on a daily basis.
8. Door mats must be recessed to avoid accidents.
9. An overhead projection at the entrance is needed for protection in inclement weather.
10. Water fountains and sinks must be accessible to wheelchair participants. (Dehydration is *very* prevalent among older people and access to water is imperative.)
11. Windows should offer an interesting view and be low enough for people who are seated to comfortably enjoy the view. (FSL files, 1983 [edited by author])

Impaired older persons attending adult day care centers have special needs which may not occur to younger or more active people who are planning a center. Older people are particularly sensitive to heat and cold. Stable air temperatures are important and each room should be free from drafts and extreme changes in temperature.

Circulation is poor among many older people, and they themselves may not recognize their own needs.

Since vision diminishes in old age, lighting should be brighter than is needed for younger people. However, glare is a problem for older people and should be minimized. Clocks, calendars, and signs should have large lettering and recent research shows that white letters on dark red, green, or black backgrounds are most easily read (Padula, 1983). The University of Michigan Institute on Gerontology has excellent audiovisual materials on this subject (University of Michigan, Michigan Media, 1981). Color coding for bathrooms, door handles, and kitchen areas often give visual cues to those experiencing problems with eyesight or disorientation. Large pictures are also helpful.

REFERRALS

Referrals to geriatric specialists (e.g., geriatric internist, geropsychiatrists, geropsychologists) should be made when a staff member needs assistance in diagnosis, treatment, and/or management of a participant. Appropriate referrals should be discussed in the weekly case meeting. Of course, some geriatric referrals depend largely upon the availability of specialists in the area, the staff's knowledge about the aging process (particularly the psychology of aging), the family's attitude, and socioeconomic status, etc., of the participant. Sources of referrals include but are not limited to social workers, psychologists, physicians, clergy, allied health, and various health care professionals (e.g., internists, psychiatrists, podiatrists, ophthalmologists, etc.).

However, prior to initiating a referral, it is advisable to note the symptoms and changes that have been observed in the participant. Talk with the participant's family or caregiver about this behavioral change. Note the duration and time of occurrence, the precipitating factors that may have contributed to the behavioral change, and the type of resolution the participant has made. After investigating the problem (carefully and sensitively), bring it to the director's attention. Then the family, the participant, the director, and the staff member will sit down to discuss the present situation. Only after the family has been included should a referral to their physician be made. All referrals should be followed up within two weeks of initiation.

INTAKE AND REVIEW PROCEDURES

FSL requires each participant to have an initial medical examination completed by a physician or clinic. A physician must provide medical clearance for program activities.

Review Procedures

1. Initial screening is completed by a registered nurse or social worker.
2. The social worker takes a social history of the participant.
3. The medical history is recorded.
4. Functional assessments are made by a registered nurse, physical therapist, and/or occupational therapist.
5. A final evaluation on program admission is completed by the multidisciplinary ADC team.
6. A treatment plan is prepared by the team.
7. An informal two-week trial is provided to each participant.
8. The participant's program is evaluated at least every six months by the treatment team.

INTERNSHIPS

Student internships in various disciplines (e.g., social work, psychology, nursing, physical and occupational therapy, art, music and drama, etc.) are encouraged by FSL. Students receive trained supervision at their field placement by appropriate staff depending on the intern's major course of study as well as the university's field placement instructor. To qualify for a field placement, a student is generally enrolled in gerontology, social work, nursing or other fields that include a practicum as part of the course of study at a local college or university, and wishes to have a field experience to complement his/her academic training. Students are interviewed and screened prior to placement both by their academic institution and the on-site supervisor.

STANDARDS AND REGULATIONS

Arizona Department of Economic Security has developed guidelines and requirements for the establishment and functioning of adult day care centers (see Appendix).

SUMMARY

Adult day care must be viewed as one service along a continuum of long-term care services as an older person moves from total independence to dependence. Adult day care has come a very long way in a short period of time. Although there are various definitions and models, adult day care is a program for the frail or infirmed elderly that is designed around individual program goals and objectives in order to help the individual remain in his/her community while maintaining as much independence as possible. As the need for alternatives in the long-term care arena grow, so will the need for an ever-increasing demand for adult day care centers, new and innovative funding resources and services, and fully staffed and trained personnel.

NOTE

1. Arizona has been the only state in the nation not to participate in the federal Medicaid program. In 1982, the Arizona legislature established the Arizona Health Care Cost Containment System (AHCCCS). Its primary purpose is to finance medical care for the indigent. AHCCCS (pronounced ACCESS), however, differs from Medicaid programs in financing, benefits, administrative arrangements, medical care, delivery structure, and provider payment principles. Currently, AHCCCS has received a waiver to eliminate certain mandatory benefits that are covered by Medicaid (e.g., no long-term care service coverage) (Arizona Statewide Health Coordinating Council, 1982).

Chapter Two

Programs, Interventions, and Strategies

There is a wide range of interventions used by adult day care centers in the treatment of the elderly and the disabled. These interventions include physical therapy, speech therapy, audiology, reality orientation, remotivation therapy, art therapy, and reminiscence therapy. Each has a special contribution to make to the well-being of the participant. For example, physical therapy helps the participant begin his/her return to independence. Speech therapy and audiology help restore communication abilities. Reality orientation is based on the principle that repeated orientations to the environment will reduce disorientation; while remotivation therapy, reminiscence therapy, art therapy, and recreational therapy are concerned with general psychosocial functioning.

The following sections will discuss FSL's primary programs: nutrition, therapies, activities, and exercises in the adult day care centers. Following each program's discussion, specific interventions, strategies, and examples will be provided.

NUTRITION

Nutrition is the science of food and its relationship to health. Proper nutrition means fulfilling the body's needs for certain elements. An adequate diet helps to prevent disease, gives energy, aids in the growth and repair of tissues, regulates the body's elimination of waste, and stimulates the appetite. The human body needs the following substances: proteins to build, repair and maintain tissues; carbohydrates to give heat and energy; vitamins and minerals to

35

maintain proper body function; and water for a healthy fluid balance to aid in the discharge of waste.

The percentage of nutritional deficiencies in geropsychiatric disorders is unknown. Research has shown that 70% of all hospitalized geriatric patients have inadequate diets. FSL recognizes the need for good nutritional diets and habits in the elderly, and nutrition is viewed as a major component of health.

FSL's adult day care clients are served one well-balanced meal at noon as well as mid-morning and mid-afternoon snacks. Participants can be provided with a therapeutic or "modified" diet on request. Nutritional counseling is provided to participants. Nutritional meals at adult day care centers are an integral part of the socializing experience for this client group. Coffee, juice, and water are provided throughout the day. Clients are encouraged to drink fluids, particularly water, to prevent dehydration (especially during the months of May through September). The Area Agency on Aging and Arizona's Department of Economic Security (DES), and its (DES') nutritionist are involved in planning meals for clients. Generally speaking, most meals are independently catered, funds are provided by the local Area Agency on Aging, and menus are approved by a DES nutritionist. Picnics, box lunches, and barbecues are also planned for special events.

THERAPIES WITH THE FRAIL PARTICIPANT

The purpose of the various therapies is generally to improve the participant's socialization and to maintain as much of their independence as possible. The staff must be able to recognize that a participant's withdrawal and isolation can exacerbate dementia and/or its symptoms. Most therapies are designed to maximize and enhance the participation of even the most severely impaired persons so that he/she can benefit from a discussion on the time of day or the weather while increasing the interaction between the older person and his/her environment.

Reality Orientation

Reality orientation, also known as "RO," is a therapeutic technique based on the assumption that repeated orientations to the environment will reduce disorientation, confusion, and withdrawal from the environment (Folsom, 1968). The efficacy of RO has been established in several studies (Barnes, 1974; Citrin & Dixon, 1977; Hanley, McGuire & Byrd, 1981; Woods, 1979). RO is an effective therapeutic intervention to use with participants who experience a moderate to severe amount of dementia. The primary symptoms of dementia include memory loss, confusion, disorientation, and poor judgment. Techniques have been developed to remedy the withdrawal and mental deterioration that accompanies this disease process in some participants (Folsom, 1966; Taulbee & Folsom, 1966). The treatment philosophy with these clients is a positive one. Goals focus on improving or maintaining cognitive functioning experienced by some participants. However, consistent evidence as to its long-term effectiveness has not been supported (Gotestam, 1980).

Reality orientation is a 24-hour process in which every contact with the participant helps them reorient or reeducate themselves. This treatment emphasizes repetition of basic day-to-day information to stimulate the individual's awareness. Reality orientation, if it is to be effective, must be the responsibility of all the staff who are in contact with the participants and their family members.

Folsom (1966) reported that RO implies a specific set of ideas to be followed. These include:

1. Strive for a calm environment.
2. Establish set routine.
3. Offer clear responses to participant's questions.
4. Speak clearly.
5. Guide participants around with clear directions.
6. Remind participants of date, time, place, etc.
7. Do not allow patients to remain confused by allowing them to ramble tangentially on in their speech and activities.
8. Be as structured as possible.
9. Be sincere.

10. Make requests of participants in a calm manner.
11. Provide consistency.

There are two parts to reality orientation: the general environment and structured classes. The participants are always addressed by their names and participants frequently are reminded of the person's name with whom they are talking. That staff member should wear a name tag. Generally the environment should have large reality-based signs, clocks, calendars, name tags, and reminders of birthdays, holidays, and activities. Structured classes should be held on a daily basis in small groups and for short periods of time.

In developing a reality orientation program for the elderly participants in adult day care many of the techniques used with brain-injured younger patients can be employed with this population. Such techniques include, but are not limited to, the following (Folsom, 1966, 1968; Mitchell, 1966):

1. Introduce yourself. Repeat your name if necessary and have participant repeat and recall your name.
2. Set a calm, friendly, and relaxed atmosphere. Speak slowly and clearly. Make sure to look directly at participants.
3. Plan simple activities initially, like a calendar book. Then after various successes, move to more complex and gratifying activities.
4. Make minimal demands on participants. Remember he/she is confused. After providing clear, simple instructions, spend as much time as possible with the participant. After leaving him/her, return frequently and give instructions.
5. Remember that social interaction with others is an important part of this program which will facilitate a return to reality and build self-esteem.
6. As the participant improves, staff may wish to have spelling sessions on simple reality-oriented words (day of week, month, city, etc.).

Folsom (1966) has observed that RO may provide very basic information. For example, participants who do not know their names are taught this crucial information. If they do not know where they are, they are told. Then they learn the day of the week, month, year, and their ages. Participants may experience disorientation for weeks and then may slowly begin to show evidence of learning and remembering past learned information. Once information is learned, the participant begins to recall other knowledge and recalls previously learned material. In essence, RO is a reeducational process utilizing repetition to stimulate participants' awareness of self and their relationship to the environment.

A relatively recent approach to RO is the use of expressive art and writing as a therapeutic tool (Weiss, 1980). This technique incorporates and integrates reality-based material that is gained over the course of a lifetime. It helps develop self-esteem and integrity by allowing participants to learn, develop, and grow from their contact in life as opposed to memorization of concepts of reality. The art and writing techniques facilitate increased orientation and a better understanding of previous achievements, problems, significant events, and conflicts, and often help to increase a participant's hopes for the future (Weiss, 1979). Art and writing RO groups are approximately one hour in length. They are held two or three times per week. A different theme is chosen at each session and discussed by the group.

At the beginning of each session, each participant is asked to fill out the short RO questionnaire (Barnes, 1974). The questionnaire is designed to test the participant's basic knowledge. When a participant is unable to write because of physical or cognitive limitations, the group leader can fill in the answers as the participant replies. The questionnaire, when completed, serves as a stimulus for group discussion and interactions. After discussing the items on the questionnaire, usually art or written expression of the topic is carried out by the participant for 15 minutes. As the group discusses the artwork or written material, the group leader reiterates reality-based information (e.g., day of the week, time, weather, special holidays, events, etc.). This reiteration helps other group members learn from the participant.

Reality-based themes provide stimulating discussions which in turn facilitate art, writing, and reminiscing which may bridge the past and present experiences of the participants. The group could last one month or continue indefinitely, during which time there should be a theme for each week to provide some structure. Brook,

Degun, and Mather (1975) pointed out that improvements in RO are attributed to a well-defined and reinforcing repetitive therapy. For example, week one could focus on living situations or homes past and present. Week two could focus on friends and relationships. Week three could focus on self-worth. All themes should be planned to have value to the participants so as to increase recall, interpersonal relations, communication, and to encourage discussion.

Another RO exercise is to select 20 items to which participants are to be oriented. At least one novel feature might relate to the participants' family, home, and neighborhood in addition to the person, place, time, and current event items. A RO board may be used as a helpful aid in implementing various exercises. A RO board that lists the name and location of the adult day care center, the date, weather, and other basic information is useful. Each participant is asked to read the information on the board. A picture of the President of the United States, a map of Arizona, and a map of the United States can be beneficial in orienting participants.

Remotivation Therapy

Remotivation therapy is a technique to restore self-worth and to encourage pleasant and positive experiences in an individual's life. Its goal is to resocialize and to facilitate activities commensurate with the individual's abilities and desires. Furthermore, the philosophy behind remotivation is that all clients have healthy untouched areas of their personality that can benefit from remotivative therapy. The general goals include developing good recall habits, stimulating and encouraging positive aspects of the personality, and developing an interest in the surrounding world. Remotivation therapy is typically used with groups that have "graduated" from reality-oriented groups.

There are five components in the remotivation program. First, the leader must create a climate of acceptance. For example, the leader should greet all participants by name and say something honest and positive about each one. Second, the leader should use pictures, family portraits, articles of interest, photographs, visual aids, and books to create ways for participants to share articles of personal interest. Third, participants should be encouraged to share their feelings, interests, and experiences, and discuss the work they used to do or historical events that have occurred during their lifetime. Fourth, participants should be encouraged to provide the group with new information or to share experiences with the others. This sharing will help to build the participant's self-worth. Fifth, the leader should create a climate of appreciation between the group members. This may be done by a smile, a touch, or a kind word to acknowledge that the time spent was enjoyable, interesting, and valuable.

The effect of dementia on group activities becomes an important consideration for the group and for the individual's behavior. For example, group leaders and volunteers should be prepared for the possibility that a demented participant may exhibit a decrease in attention and interest span, an increase in anxiety, an increase in agitation, and an increase in restlessness. These behaviors may require close supervision and flexibility.

Life Review and Reminiscence Therapy

Reminiscing and life review are important activities for the elderly. This therapy allows the participants to survey aspects of their past and may help them achieve a new and significant meaning toward life. Life review is a personal, self-evaluative form of reminiscence with intrapersonal and interpersonal dimensions (Molinari & Reichlin, 1984-1985). Butler (1963) defined life review as a "naturally occurring, universal mental process characterized by the progressive return to consciousness of past experience . . . prompted by the realization of approaching dissolution and death, and the inability to maintain one's sense of personal invulnerability." Butler (1974) further stated that life review is usually prompted by the elderly person becoming aware of his/her closeness to death. Unlike thinking about the past, as in reminiscing, life review uses memories to get some "closure" on the participant's life, particularly the difficult aspects.

McMahon and Rhudrick (1964) and LoGerfo (1980) point out three types of reminiscences:

1. Storytelling or informative reminiscence, which enhances self-esteem and the social function of oral history.
2. Reminiscence that provides material for life review.
3. Defensive or obsessive reminiscence, which is associated with guilt over negative life review or as a defense against an ungratifying present.

Part of the process of life review is conflict, in which the participant struggles through his or her failures, disappointments, and losses (Molinari & Reichlin, 1984-1985).

Reminiscence can have positive and negative values. Pincus (1970) reported several positive aspects of reminiscing, including reinforcing an individual identity, grief resolution, available material for continued life review, and coping with specific stressful experiences. Therefore, past thoughts or memories may offer psychological comfort to an older unhappy participant with his/her present situation. Moreover, the ability to look closely at oneself, one's family, one's generation and cohorts may help to restore self-worth, self-confidence, and enhance one's self-concept. Other investigators have noted some negative aspects of reminiscing, including living in the past, experiencing loneliness, avoiding new experiences, and clinging to a previous younger identity (Lewis & Butler, 1974).

Of course, there are various applicable intervention strategies that the group leader can use. Leaders can employ art, life review therapy (Zeiger, 1976), movement therapy, reminiscence (Sandel, 1978), and life history (Meyerhoff & Tufte, 1975) in most adult day care activities. Two suggestions follow: discuss mementoes that the participants have collected over time. The sharing of and discussion about these mementoes may generate solidarity and may help participants come to terms with personal aspects of their past. Discuss a personal historical event the group has each shared (e.g., the Depression, World War I, World War II) and let them reminisce about their experiences. Ideally, the group participants should form their own "community" and should develop a sense of pride for their age group (Ebersole, 1978).

The group facilitator must be knowledgeable about the various therapeutic techniques or interventions, but should also focus on the organization, structure, support, and guidance of the group. These characteristics/qualifications are usually rendered to the group by the concern, the actively involved presence, and the availability of the leader. An indirect and direct message that should be projected by the leader is the need for the group members to feel encouragement by the leader when attending group as well as when sharing and expressing themselves.

Generally, reminiscence and life review groups are ongoing, cohesive, and closed-ended (new members are not to be added during the course of the program). Within each group, unique strategies need to be employed when confronted with repetitive stories from one participant, overt sadness or crying, physical discomfort, and sensory deprivation. With repetitive data, the group leader may wish to use some diversional techniques by asking for elaboration or simply stating that the group has heard the story many times before, but the group would enjoy hearing about an event that occurred prior to the event. When reminiscing, participants may cry while sharing a personal event in their pasts, particularly when inhibitions are lowered by the trust that has built up in a closed-ended group. The leader should provide guided reminiscing, allow participants to cry, and then, in a sensitive manner, direct their sadness to a warm and caring time (e.g., was there someone during your time of sadness that made you feel better?).

In open-ended reminiscence and life review groups, newcomers are allowed to join the group at any time. Special attention by the group leader(s) should be given in order to welcome the newcomers as well as the longtime members. Moreover, the leader will need to repeat and review past programs and materials. New members as well as longtime members will benefit from the review process, and as a result, the need for information varies accordingly (Middleton, 1984).

Before beginning a reminiscence group, make certain to take care of major concerns of participants (e.g., hunger, toileting, discussion of illnesses or ailments, etc.). No group should be so goal-oriented that the participants' needs are neglected. Sensory integration or stimulation (auditory, tactile, olfactory, kinesthetic, proprioceptive, vestibule, and visual) should be added to the environment. Music should be chosen to fit the participants' expressed desires rather than the leader's needs. Usually there is no significant decline in olfactory sensors. Smells may produce various surprises and may stimulate memories. Visual materials should be bright, colorful, and large. Remember to provide participants with sufficient time to integrate material so they do not become overloaded with experiences (see Table 1).

TABLE 1 "Common Geriatric Problems and Helpful Activities"

Difficulty	Goal	Activities	Comments
(1) Short Attention Span; Poor Memory	Prevent further loss; increase use of memory in daily activities; increase ability to make simple decisions	Simple memory games (matching shapes, colors, names to faces) to advanced activities that require time management	Requires carefully structured activities, repetitive procedures, carefully graded activities that move step by step in difficulty; narrow range of choices; structured environment free of unnecessary supplies
(2) Confusion and Disorientation	Increase awareness of person, place, time and current events	Reference to familiar or necessary things in environment; e.g., parts of body; identify objects from a bag or pictures; work on simple puzzles, have participant use complete sentences	Need to give written and verbal instructions. Large calendars and clocks. Staff member wear large print name tag
(3) Wandering, Unable to sit still	Direct to safe activity	Short-term well structured activity; gross motor activities	Supervision required with tools and equipment
(4) Inappropriate behavior (by crying, laughing when there's no justification	Help participant gain control over behavior	May need to move participant to quieter activity without distracting attention of others	Crying inappropriately may indicate sadness or it may be indicative of a symptom of Organic Brain Syndrome (OBS)
(5) Inability to communicate basic needs	Increase verbal or non-verbal behavior	Activities mentioned in #2	If Non-OBS, refer to speech therapist and carry out prescribed activities
(6) Disruptive behavior (cursing, anger, outburst of emotions)	Stop disruptive behavior and help show participant appropriate behavior	After responding appropriately, "I can see you are unhappy," ... disturbed ... Shift to a quiet activity or one that participant can "work off" emotions	There might be a disturbance in the participant's home life or environment
(7) Limited use of joints	Maintain or increase strength and range of motion in affected area	Repetitive, graded steps for fine and gross motor activities	Pay attention to the "whole" person

HEALTH SERVICES

Health surveillance is also a key service in any adult day care center. An adult day care program does not usually include direct medical care, diagnosis, or treatment. However, continual health surveillance occurs in most adult day care centers. Monitoring blood pressure, pulse, and weight is performed monthly. Daily health services include assisting clients, when necessary, with medications. In accordance with the purpose of adult day care in helping each individual maintain maximum independence, adult day care participants, when possible, are encouraged to take and be responsible for their own medications.

Each participant's personal physician and the adult day care center's nurse try to work together to coordinate the participant's health care. A medical form is filled out before any participant starts attending the center and is updated when any change takes place. The center's nurse also provides health education on an individual and a group basis. The nurse also coordinates any physical, speech, occupational, or recreational therapy that takes place at the center.

Physical Therapy

Physical therapy is the use of physical means to reduce pain and maintain or improve physical functions. The goal of physical therapy focuses on maintaining, improving, or restoring the function of the neuromusculoskeletal, pulmonary, and cardiovascular systems through physical intervention. Common disorders that benefit from physical therapy may include arthritis, amputations, neurological problems, and orthopedics.

The aim of physical therapy is two-fold. First, physical therapy improves the participant's restorative potential. Second, services are a necessary management technique to use with a specific disability. Objectives include: providing active and passive exercises to increase strength, endurance, coordination and range of motion; facilitating activities needed in daily living; stimulating motor activities and learning; and applying physical agents to relieve pain or alter physiologic status.

Physical therapy can be a part of the adult day care participant's therapeutic regimen if requested by a physician and implemented by a physical therapist. Physical therapy can also be viewed as a continuum of care beginning with prevention, screening, crisis intervention, short-term and long-term rehabilitation, and ending with maintenance in a long-term situation.

Exercise

Being physically fit for the adult day care participant means being able to do things they need or want to do in their daily lives. One of the benefits of fitness is the sense of independence and self-esteem it provides. Some of the benefits of exercise include:

1. An increase in lung function.
2. A reduction in irritability.
3. A lower heart rate.
4. A greater blood flow which will keep kidneys and other organs functioning.
5. The maintenance of a fat/lean ratio in the body composition.
6. An increased interest in the surrounding world.
7. An increased energy and vigor in daily activities.
8. An increased mental functioning and emotional stability.
9. A decrease in anxiety and depression.

The impact of exercise will, of course, depend upon the type of exercise program, the frequency of exercise, and the participant's attitude and motivation to maximize his/her life. Typically, functional decline that seems to be associated with age is actually due to a lack of exercise and can be reversed through therapeutic exercise programs. FSL's adult day care program provides the opportunity to prevent or reverse a large portion of functional decline many individuals associate with aging.

A preliminary examination is necessary. The type of exercise is as important as the intensity level of the exercise. Exercise programs for older people should maximize the rhythmic activity of large muscle masses. Such exercises include walking, jogging, running, and swimming. Moreover, for muscle tone maintenance, isometric exercises have been of interest lately as well as isotonic exercises that are more active and go through a full range of motion (Pardini, 1984).

Range of motion (ROM) exercises are described as the full extent of movement in a body joint. Normal ROM is the ability to perform full movement of a joint. Functional ROM is less than the normal ability to move a body joint, but with enough ability to permit the participant to perform activities of daily living. Activities of daily living are movements that a participant does as a part of his/her daily self-care routine.

ROM exercises must be scheduled in regular and frequent intervals twice a day, five days a week. General guidelines for therapists include engaging the participant in active exercise when possible, following up suggestions recommended by the physician, moving each joint through a full range of motion, observing degrees of fatigue, instructing the participant to carry out exercises independently, checking on the participant to see if exercises are being carried out properly, and discontinuing exercise motions if pain or resistance is evident.

The four types of ROM exercises that may benefit the geriatric participant are free, resistive, passive, and active.

1. Free active ROM exercises are carried out solely by the participant.
2. Resistive ROM exercises are done by the participant against a pull provided by another person or machine.
3. Active-assistance ROM exercises are done in part by the participant and in part by another individual or machine.
4. Passive ROM exercises are done to a participant by another person or by a machine without the help of the participant.

Participants are reevaluated at regular intervals and their exercise program is adjusted to meet individual needs. Reevaluation includes the following:

Endurance. (a) Cardiovascular — Improving the endurance of the heart, the circulation, and the lungs may be *the* most important component of physical fitness. Aerobic exercise includes any activity of the large muscles, performed repetitively and rhythmically for 15-30 minutes, three times a week, preferably every other day. Cardiovascular (CV) endurance usually reduces fatigue, increases energy, and reduces risks associated with CV disease. (b) Muscular —

Endurance is the length of time particular muscles can sustain an activity like walking, holding heavy objects, or maintaining good posture. Carrying groceries and lifting objects are activities of daily living that require forearm, shoulder, and back muscle endurance. Muscle endurance is also produced by jogging, aerobics, walking, swimming, and other aerobic activities.

Muscle strength. Muscle strength is the amount of force that can be exerted by a contraction of a muscle. Some activities of daily living that require muscle strength are lifting groceries, taking out garbage, and coping with household emergencies. Shoulder and back strength are needed for good posture. Exercises like isometrics, isokinetics, weight training, and some calisthenics help develop muscle strength.

Flexibility. This is important to all major bodily joints to improve movement and to avoid muscle pulls, strains, injuries, and low back pain. To improve flexibility, range of motion exercises that exercise each joint should be conducted, coupled with slow stretching exercises, repeated consistently and regularly.

Coordination and agility. Coordination is the ability to organize physical activity in skillful movement and to coordinate different actions of each other with the ego. Agility is the ability to coordinate movements and change directions quickly and safely. Swimming provides the best exercise for arm/leg coordination, dancing for coordination and agility, and golf for eye-hand-foot coordination and agility.

Occupational Therapy

Purposeful activity is described as the trademark of occupational therapy. Various researchers have reported a relationship between occupational therapy (OT) and the prevention of isolation, boredom, and preoccupation with problems when accompanied by high activity and high life satisfaction in the elderly (Hasselkaus & Kiernat, 1973; Nystron, 1974; Warren, 1977). Occupational therapy may be defined as "any activity, mental or physical, definitely prescribed and guided for the distinct purpose of contributing to and hastening recovery from disease or injury" (Dunton & Licht, 1950). Furthermore, other researchers have indicated that occupational therapy contributes to the physical, psychological, social, and economic rehabilitation of the participant.

The role of the occupational therapist usually consists of administrating and interpreting tests and clinical observations used for evaluating fine- and gross-motor control, sensiomotor integration levels, perceptual-motor performance, new developmental states, and the participant's abilities in performing activities of daily living (Langdon & Langdon, 1983). With demented participants, the occupational therapist should approach each session with the participant as if it were a first meeting (unless the therapist observes some recognition from the participant). Habitual activities learned early in life as well as overlearned activities may be more successful than completely new ones.

Occupational therapy may include community outings to evaluate functional abilities and provide the opportunity for participants to practice activities outside the adult day care center. Activities should provide the participant with the opportunity for maintaining good habits and appearance, the opportunity to exercise all talents, and sufficient physical exercises of help with mobility (MacDonald, 1964). For women, some activities may include preparing meals and cooking, knitting, crocheting, and mending. For men, simple woodwork and gardening may be enjoyed.

Recreational Therapy

Recreational therapy is an intervention described by Kraus (1978) and Carter, Van Andel, and Robb (1985) as a means of strengthening aspects of the individual, enabling him/her to maximize existing potentials in the face of limitations, and to prevent other disabilities and disorders. Its purpose is to encourage self-respect, stimulate physical and mental abilities, decrease symptoms of physical and mental regression due to illness, and provide a way of preventing depression and feelings of hopelessness.

In recreational therapy, part of the focus is to shift attention and feelings away from the participants' illnesses and losses to living in the present. The process may be community or residentially-based. Most community-based programs focus on the educational or supportive role of recreation whereas the others emphasize rehabilitation and preventive goals (Carter et al., 1985). Recreation with the elderly provides benefits such as improving physical health, improving emotional well-being, reawakening creative impulses, encouraging social involvement, providing meaningful roles, and offering a threshold to other social services (Kraus, 1978).

Recreational therapy is usually implemented through FSL's activity programs. Recreational programs include, but are not limited to: creative projects; intellectual stimulation; social activities and interactions; exercises; and spiritual and/or religious activities, programs or events. These activities may be presented individually or in a group setting.

ACTIVITIES

The value of activity for the elderly has been well-documented in the gerontological literature. One of the most significant contributions derived from aerospace research has been the effect of sensory deprivation on cognitive functioning (Galton, 1979). When elderly people are not exposed to normal or complex sensory stimulation (i.e., sounds, tastes, touch, auditory stimuli) within the environment, they may become vulnerable to disorganized thinking for a short period of time.

The causes of sensory deprivation are varied. A decrease in visual or auditory acuity may impair a participant's reality testing. As a result of this decrement, many elderly participants have become ostracized from their social environment. This ostracization results in increased tension, agitation, and depression while negatively affecting sensory deficits on the part of the participant.

The goal of all FSL adult day care activity programs is to keep participants involved, interested, and as active as possible in day-to-day living. FSL's adult day care participants have the opportunity to learn as well as the opportunity to gain a fuller social, recreational, and nutritional life. In short, FSL strives to promote "good health" in the elderly.

FSL's adult day care activities include field trips, lectures, classes, and expressive activities. Sometimes learning is combined with social and recreational experiences such as drama, theatre programs, concerts, games, parties, and other social events.

Structured daily activities should be consistent, predictable (with respect to occurrence), and sufficiently diverse. This combination of factors is crucial in providing diversion, stimulation, and in helping to develop the clients' full potentials. Activities should not be limited to "bingo" games; begin to prepare other relevant activities that can provide enjoyment and build self-confidence and self-worth. Remember: HOW A SERVICE IS OFFERED IS JUST AS IMPORTANT AS WHAT IS OFFERED!

FSL strives for a quality activity program that enhances individuality and contributes to the participants' quality of care. The following pages will review a number of activities that have been implemented in adult day care centers in Arizona and other parts of the country.

INTERGENERATIONAL ACTIVITIES

Grandparenthood is a role that is universally available to approximately 4/5 of people over the age of 65 (Butler & Lewis, 1982). Benedek (1970) has described grandparenthood as a time when "the stresses and responsibilities of parenting are removed and a time to enjoy their grandchildren more than they enjoyed their own children." Grandparents project hope and tend to be indulgent to their grandchildren. Their love is not burdened by parental doubts and anxieties as it was when their own children were young.

Some investigators (Kahana & Kahana, 1970; Butler & Lewis, 1982) have studied grandparenthood from a grandchild's perspective. Positive feelings and regard toward grandparents tend to be associated with the amount of contact, grandparent's behavior toward them, and the child's perception of older people in general and grandparents in particular. Furthermore, young children seem to appreciate a grandparent who brings them gifts, does favors, and displays open affection toward them. Older children, on the other hand, prefer sharing activities and mutual fun and activities.

Some older persons have successfully been surrogate grandparents through the Foster Grandparent program (a component of Action) or through the Adopt-a-Grandparent program. The Adopt-a-Grandparent program can begin in any adult day care center by having the social worker and/or activity coordinator, for example, plan a program with a nearby elementary school class, a church group, or children's organization. Visits should be scheduled on a regular basis (at least once a week) and each child should be encouraged to personally interact with the senior. Both children and seniors should be briefed in this activity and be helped to understand what they might expect from the visit. Some programs have found that the pairing of two children with one grandparent works best. In that way, there is a backup in case of illness and for mutual support. It is important to carefully match the children and their personality with the most appropriate grandparent. Many of the Adopt-a-Grandparent program's participants have illustrated that such programs create an openness not always found in adult relationships and may bring a positive, warm, and loving time to the youngster and the senior (Larronde, 1983).

COMPANION ANIMALS

The human/animal relationship exhibited by the elderly and their pets can provide companionship, substitute for close interpersonal relationship, enhance health status, increase opportunity for sensory stimulation, increase emotional support and a sense of well-being, lower blood pressure, and decrease medication levels (Wilson & Netting, 1983; Robb & Stegman, 1983; Levinson, 1972, 1978). Pets have become so important to the medical and psychological professions that the term "pet-facilitated psychotherapy" (PFP) has evolved. PFP is used in group environments and various long-term care facilities as adjuncts to more traditional treatments.

Dogs, cats, and birds are primarily being prescribed by doctors to older persons, particularly those who are isolated or live alone. Therapeutic effects of human/companion animal contacts have indicated that the presence of companion animals helps to serve as a conversational piece, a free zone that stimulates interactions between the participant, the pet, and other people (Corson et al., 1976; Mugford & M'Comisky, 1975). Increased interactions serve to build rapport because the pet facilitates trust, enhances communication, and diverts negative behavior. Having a pet to care for may restore dignity, minimize loneliness and prolong life (Brickel, 1979; Silden, 1983).

GAMES

Often times, the social, emotional, and physical losses experienced by the frail elderly can increase their risk of sensory deprivation. The incidence of perceptual and sensory losses on the frail elderly seem to be correlated with life satisfaction. A possible form of recreation that may promote communication between participants and staff of adult day care centers and other long-term care facilities includes "Games of Rapport" such as "Angels and Devils," "Owls and Weasels," "Roles," "Justification," "Alternatives," and "Brain and Numbskull" (Corbin & Nelson, 1980).

The board game, "Angels and Devils," resembles the marketed game "Chutes and Ladders," in its format. Player movement is accomplished by the throwing of the dice, except in the instances when a player lands on designated "sliding spaces." Sliding spaces are designated by color, design and messages. If a player lands on a sliding space, he/she selects a card from the appropriate stack and reads a behavior description. Each card which is designated by an angel or a devil on the front and on the back is a descriptive behavior that is to be read and carried out. It has been shown that interaction between participants has been quite spirited, particularly as they recollected past events in their home and alternately denied or accepted attributions of the "angel" or the "devil" cards (Corbin & Nelson, 1980).

There are also educational games that have been designed to help groups, families or individuals deal with decisions regarding the aging process. The "Family and Friends" game helps provide a better understanding of family dynamics and decision-making processes in late life (Oregon State University Extension Service, 1983). The players analyze specific situations, assess their attitudes and values, and give insight into the behavior of family members so as to consider how decisions will affect the family. Thirty to 90 minutes is needed to achieve optimum benefit from the game. Discussion following the game is encouraged, permits further skill-building, and provides a nonthreatening approach for members to express their concerns, fears, anxieties, and questions about older relatives, older persons, and themselves.

Computer Games

The elderly need stimulating challenges to their thinking processes, exercises (especially hand-eye coordination), and opportunities to enhance self-esteem by learning new material (Butler & Lewis, 1973; Solomon, 1982). The area of memory training is extremely important for many elderly. The computer is now another means by which the elderly may develop their skills and thinking processes. Its adaptable, repetitive, user-friendly, nonjudgmental approach is well-suited for helping participants with mild to moderate memory loss. Adult day care participants can have the opportunity to play a new and exciting game which provides a new means of learning logic and various methods of thinking.

The most successful games are those that can be programmed so that participants can begin at a level that is easily mastered and then progress in small increments to more advanced levels as the participant improves. The visual symbols must be well-defined and the auditory clues must be clear and distinct. Bernie Benson (of Washington State's Apple Pi Club) adapted three games to be tested among the elderly in a nursing home. His adaptations included slowing the games down, making the figures larger, and reducing the number and complexity of the visual characters. The results indicated that all of the participants who played the games reported having an enjoyable time. One person, for example, said, "Wait till I tell my son that I know how to work a computer!" Having access to a computer made those elderly people feel as though they were participating in the age of technology.

Apple Corporation has Apple II video games that can be adapted for the elderly. Brick House, Ribbet, and Country Driver are three examples of games that have been adapted for the elderly (Weisman, 1983). Atari and Intellivision also have several games that can be played at a participant's own pace.

Bingo

Bingo is a game that requires a minimum of interactions for participants who are unable to interact or develop friendships easily. It enables the activity therapist to evaluate and intervene in a participant's problem area(s) like letter reversals, inability to read, varied handicaps due to arthritis, and/or a decrease in visual/manual dexterity. Moreover, some participants gain confidence in their ability to play bingo, become more productive, and begin to enjoy other activities.

THERAPEUTIC DANCE MOVEMENT

Movement may be one of the keys to successful aging. Without movement an individual's muscles become weak and that individual may lose the ability to walk or carry out daily activities.

Dance therapy is an effective treatment for individuals with a wide variety of physical and mental difficulties. It is the use of rhythmic movement as a means of self-expression and communication that aids in the integration of the mind and the body. Particularly with the elderly, sessions encourage the participants to discover the pleasure in moving and in using energy and space. The therapeutic value of dance and movement programs increases mobility of body parts, reduces stress, and increases relaxation and socialization. Movement or dance can also modify a participant's mood and stimulate sensory awareness (Fersh, 1980).

The selection of dance movements and music depend upon participants' ethnicity, culture, physical and mental abilities, past experiences, and religious preferences. Dance or movement themes that deal with seasons, holidays, and other techniques used in remotivation and reality orientation can be effective stimulators of mental functioning. Dance and movement therapy with elderly people can help them open up to new horizons and experiences and possibly facilitate their motivation to embrace life.

MUSIC THERAPY

Music therapy is the use of musical activities to alter nonmusical behavior (Palmer, 1980). Music is a nonthreatening therapeutic tool that is also nonverbal in its form of communication. Music is a part of everyone's experience, and the elderly find it pleasurable and often challenging.

In working with the disoriented participant, the music therapist may wish to reinforce reality-based concepts of person, place, and time by actively involving the participant in a music session. For example, the therapist may play nostalgic songs of the past. The participant may recall events of the past and begin to make associations about the present. Mental processes are stimulated in a relaxing and enjoyable setting. Participants who could not be reached by any other form of communication have been reached by music. Music acts as a morale booster not only for the participants but for the staff as well.

In order to successfully reach the geriatric patient, music must be meaningful. Two types of programming have been useful: old nostalgic songs and ethnic or cultural music. Popular music during the early part of the 20th century — like jazz — was much simpler sounding than the music of today. The elderly recall "the good ole days" when life was simpler for them and their values were not so complex. Musical instruments that have special appeal to the elderly are the piano and the violin (Kartman, 1980).

Music therapy should take place at least once a week for one hour. Nostalgic music played on the piano should make for some great sing-alongs. Even nonverbal participants can respond on a "feeling" level.

When holidays approach, the holiday should be discussed with the group and appropriate music should be played on the piano. Holidays may be included in a musical reality-orientation session. For example, for the Fourth of July songs could be played such as "America the Beautiful," the "Star Spangled Banner," and "Yankee Doodle Dandy." Also "musical memory" programs have been effective morale builders which have a powerful impact on the participants.

ART THERAPY

Art therapy provides the opportunity for full expression of emotions and thoughts. Introducing art, however, to the geriatric participant must be done in a nonthreatening, noncompetitive, and tactful manner. A trusting and warm emotional climate should be provided. The goal of a therapeutic art program is to stimulate changes in or bring about stability for elderly participants.

Activities should strive to accommodate each participant's physical, psychological, and social needs. Art activities should be relevant and meaningful to their daily social lives. Art therapy allows even the confused participant another means of communicating. Supervision and planning of an art project is a must. The disoriented participant will require more structure. For example, masking tape may be used to mark off the area in which each participant paints. Make a sample of the finished product. Before the activity, modify any procedures and complete any portions that must be done by staff.

CRAFTS

Crafts can help rebuild the participant's self-esteem that may have been previously diminished through loss of income, loss of roles, and loss of health. Some activities require cutting or tearing, gluing, and applying a finish. Decoupage, papier-mache, and tissue-paper collage are activities that require very little coordination. Although the activities are structured crafts, they all contain an imaginative component in the selection and placement of materials – all good group projects. Cutting is a good activity for strengthening the muscles that open and close the hand. If precision cutting is required, a paper cutter or a geriatric aide could accommodate. For those who cannot cut with scissors, another participant may lend a hand. Suggested crafts include:

Decoupage. Decoupage can be used to encourage gross-motor coordination. The repetitive nature of sanding and/or pounding is good for the elderly individuals who have difficulty initiating motion or who have limited fine-motor coordination. Tool handlers and "C" clamps can be used to help give a better grasp of the wood. This is also a good activity for those who have a visual or perceptual disability.

Papier-Mache. Papier-Mache consists primarily of tearing and/or cutting strips of paper and placing them (layering or overlapping) on a smooth surface. Minimal gross-motor coordination, muscle strength, and/or visual acuity is needed to complete this activity. The thickness of the paper being torn can be varied to make the project adaptable for strengthening muscles. Tearing paper can be a good way of venting frustration and/or aggression.

Make certain to carefully choose projects that have some degree of sophistication (e.g., do not try to teach something that you cannot do well yourself) and purpose. You might also want to show the completed project at the beginning of this activity.

Tissue Paper Collage. Tissue paper collage requires some dexterity in picking up the thin pieces of tissue. However, utilizing the overlap method eliminates the need for precise placement. Tissue paper can be used with Elmer's glue, water, and paintbrush. With a water and glue mixture, have participant brush the mixture onto the cardboard. Other smooth materials (leaves, flowers, etc.) can be glued onto a collage as well as textured materials such as beads, buttons, rice, noodles, bark, and eggshells.

Printing and Stationery. Printing is an activity all participants enjoy. Techniques vary from using hand-cut blocks to elaborate silk screening. Some coordination and grasp strength is needed. Placing the block to the side of the participant encourages reaching as well as flexion and extension of the elbow. The vegetables and blocks may be cut by staff members if participants are limited in ability. The printing can be done, however, by the frail elderly.

Other Craft Projects. Below is a brief list of other craft projects appropriate for FSL's adult day care participants.

1. Papier-mache — mash method
2. Magazine page art
3. Printing and stationery
    a. Printing with styrofoam
    b. Leaf prints
4. Stitchery
    a. Embroidery
    b. Needlepoint
    c. Knitting
    d. Crocheting
5. Tie dying
6. Decorative curtains
7. Art (including computer graphics)
8. Mosaics
9. Use of clay
10. Sand terrarium and sand cradle

11. Horticulture (including vegetable gardening)

Many of these activities provide visual rather than tactile stimulation. Psychologically, these types of activities (repetitive motion, scrawling crayons) meet the needs of participants who have a short attention span, are limited in physical condition and have difficulty following precise instructions and movements. Additionally, good social interactions are usually created during participation because a great deal of sharing is constantly going on in the group.

The goal of art is to enjoy oneself. Introduce participants to paint and brushes, and let them cover a paper with thick and thin brush strokes. Encourage their practice of folding paper. Select various themes for art or painting projects such as color compositions, visual awareness, and peripheral associations (i.e., red equals roses, fire, etc.; blue equals sky, water).

SUMMARY

The issues addressed in this chapter were concerned with reviewing various programs, interventions, and strategies for effective service delivery of adult day care. Numerous researchers have reported that as elderly people age, maintaining them in the home becomes an increasingly important issue. Home seems to play a significant part in one's identity, familiarity, and autonomy. Issues involving concerns about support services, respite, safety, and socialization for an older person continue to arise and are prominent themes for the elderly and caregivers.

Adult day care is designed to assist moderately impaired, frail, or handicapped elderly to maintain or restore their independence and living status. It is just one of many long-term care services. Programs can offer medical care, health screening, individual/group/family psychotherapy, counseling, occupational therapy, physical therapy, educational/recreational/leisure activities, meals/nutritional counseling, and plenty of opportunities for socializing. It provides a pleasant, comfortable, and safe environment for many isolated, "home bound" elderly. Adult day care programs generally strive to promote optimum physical and mental health through various therapeutic programs.

Chapter Three

Foundation for Senior Living
Operations Manual

The operations manual explains every phase of the adult day care business. It describes the services that are performed in the adult day care centers and it contains samples of all forms and reports necessary for operating a center. During the training program that is offered to a person selected to operate an adult day care center, he/she will be provided an operations manual along with specific training for operating a center, instructions for filling out all forms and reports, and directions for effectively marketing the program locally.

The operations manual is designed to be placed in a loose-leaf notebook. The pages are numbered consecutively. When changes are made in policy, price, or method, the corporate office sends a revised page to each center with instructions to remove and throw away the outdated page. Listed below is an outline of the Foundation for Senior Living's operations manual:

A. Adult Day Care Statement of Purpose
B. Routine Daily Procedures
C. Operational Procedures
D. Cleaning Routines
E. Bookkeeping Procedures
F. Social Services
G. Health Surveillance
H. Activities
I. Volunteers
J. Personal Hygiene
K. Monthly Reports and Forms

The following pages provide a description of many items contained in the Foundation for Senior Living's Adult Day Care operations manual.

STATEMENT OF PURPOSE (Appendix A)

In order to maintain a high standard of care throughout the network of adult day care centers operated by the Foundation for Senior Living, it is imperative that all personnel understand the purpose of the operation. The statement of purpose defines the terms of adult day care and lists the services provided, the target population that is served, the philosophy of treatment, and the general cost of the service.

DAILY ROUTINE PROCEDURES (Appendix B)

Opening the Center (Appendix B1)

Standardized procedures for opening and closing the center and serving lunch and snacks are important for safety, program monitoring, cost control, liability, and billing. Opening the center involves unlocking the center and taking care of the physical plant, such as adjusting thermostats, lights, etc. This is the first activity of the day, and the person responsible for this prepares the building for the day's activities.

Contribution envelopes are placed on a table just inside the entrance to the center. These are for voluntary donations by clients and are very important to the overall general operating budget. To increase donations, envelopes are attached to each person's name badge as a reminder. Each center collects between $500 and $4,000 a month in client donations.

Sign-in sheets are placed on the same table along with the donation envelopes and name tags. The daily sign-in sheet enables center staff to keep track of the time each participant arrives at the center and when he/she leaves. This sheet is used for billing purposes, as clients are charged by the hour. In addition, it lets the staff know which clients are present that day. Several times during the day the staff will count the number of participants present to ensure that no one has wandered away or left the center without proper supervision.

Name tags are worn all day by clients and staff members. The client's name, center, and telephone number of the center are written on the name badge. Name badges are worn to aid the participants and staff in getting to know one another, assist those with memory losses in communicating, and are a safety precaution should anyone wander away from the center.

Several lists and schedules need to be reviewed daily. This includes the snack menu, along with the daily sign-in sheet, so that proper substitutions can be prepared for people on special diets. The monthly activity schedule also needs to be checked each morning to prepare for any special events taking place. If any visitors are expected that day, their names should be written in the communication book to inform all staff members (see Appendix C11). Finally, the volunteer schedule listing the names of people scheduled to volunteer should be checked so that name tags and assignments can be prepared before they arrive at the center.

The staff communication book is a loose-leaf notebook. Anything that is not part of the everyday routine (e.g., if a staff person calls in sick, if any visitors are expected, or if the van is going in the shop to be repaired) is noted. The notebook should be kept in a centralized location, and it is the responsibility of each staff member to read the book before beginning the day's work. The person responsible for opening the center is responsible for seeing that the book is in its proper place at the beginning of each day.

Another duty of the person opening the center is to make coffee for the day. This includes placing the cups, cream, and sugar in the service area. The staff member opening the center must also check the restrooms to make sure there is an adequate supply of paper products and soap. During the day the staff will be very busy, and each morning is the logical time to stock, refill, or replace supplies.

The person opening the center is also responsible for placing the luncheon sign-in sheet in its assigned location. Each client is required to sign-in during the lunch period. This is very important as it is another check to ensure that everyone who is supposed to be there is, and that no one has wandered away. Another reason for asking participants to sign their names a total of three times during the day is to encourage independence. Many disabled people have little or no responsibility for their lives, and may never be required to write their name. This gives them back some responsibility for themselves, albeit ever so small.

Greeting Routine (Appendix B2)

When clients arrive at the center each morning, it is extremely important that they are made to feel important, needed, and that they belong. Many participants initially feel anxious and unsure of where they are going when beginning adult day care. It is vital for the staff to make each person feel comfortable and a part of the center. For clients who have been attending for some time, it is important to treat them with the same enthusiasm as the new participants in the program.

A staff member should meet the van or car and assist the driver with unloading the participants and assist them in walking into the center. The driver is on a very tight schedule and needs assistance — particularly when loading and unloading participants.

As a participant enters the center, they should be greeted warmly. As each staff member gets to know each participant, a handshake or a hug will occur naturally. Each person must be comfortable in expressing their warmth and affection in their own way. Time will dictate which approach is best for each individual.

As noted earlier, each participant should be encouraged to sign their name on the daily sign-in sheet and note the time they arrived at the center. At this point, each participant should be assisted in putting their name tag on. Many participants feel that adult day care is their place of work, and they enjoy putting their name tag on at the beginning of each day. One way of making new participants feel welcome on their first day in the program is to have their name tags ready for them to wear. They should always be asked what they prefer to be called (i.e., Mrs. Smith, Mildred, Millie, etc.).

Each morning participants should be encouraged to get their own cup of coffee. To increase the independence of each individual, it is important whenever possible for clients to pour their own coffee, carry it back to where they will drink it, and take care of the empty cup when they are finished.

Any pertinent information, including any physical changes of the participants' conditions, should be reported to the nurse or director and recorded in the staff communications book. When a participant calls in sick, this should be noted on the daily sign-in sheet (see Appendix B7).

Snacks (Appendix B3)

Health regulations require each person who assists in food preparation — including participants — to have a food handler's permit.

Snacks are provided mid-morning and mid-afternoon. Snacks promote socialization, add to good nutrition, and help prevent dehydration (life-threatening for people living in the Southwest). Snacks, prepared with the help of a few of the participants, consist of fruit, juices, cheese, toast, cereal, etc. Substitutions are made for participants on diabetic diets, and all meals are prepared with no added salt for those on a low-sodium diet.

As the emphasis on maximizing each individual's independence is promoted throughout the day, the staff will encourage each participant to serve him/herself and help others who cannot (see Appendix B3.3).

Lunch (Appendix B4)

It has been found that catered meals are less costly, provide better variety, and are easier to manage when operating an adult day care center. While lunchtime is the focal point of the day, the meal itself is often secondary to the opportunity for socialization among the participants. It is common for elderly people to suffer sensory losses, including a decrease in their taste sensations. In addition, they may be suffering from poor nutrition and possible dehydration. These two problems alone can be causes for memory loss and mental health problems. Once the person begins eating properly and drinking enough fluids, their physical health and mental well-being improves. If a participant says he/she doesn't feel like eating, he/she will usually eat with others who are enjoying their food and are involved in a stimulating conversation. Using round tables instead of long rectangular tables promotes conversation, further encouraging participants to eat.

Participants need to be encouraged to help set the table and to clean up afterwards. Many frail elderly people have lost the opportunity to feel useful. By allowing them to wash and set the tables, it gives each participant who helps the feeling of purpose and useful activity. Placemats, tables, and plates should be in contrasting colors. For people with visual problems, a light-surfaced table with a white placemat, plate, and lightcolored food is not only unappetizing, but very hard to distinguish. Food should be placed attractively on the plates using foods with different colors and textures for variation.

One-third of the daily nutritional requirement, as directed by the federal government, should be served. To keep food costs at a minimum, proper portion control is a must. However, some individuals' needs — which must be met — are more than the minimum daily requirement. Conversely, others may be overwhelmed by the amount of food that must be served to meet the federal guideline. For the latter, serving small portions from the required amount to a second plate is suggested. As each portion is eaten, additional small servings are given until the minimum required amount of food has been taken. This procedure also works well with disoriented persons who are often confused with large amounts of food. Another hint for clients who may be unable to handle utensils is to provide appropriate finger food such as slices of cheese, fruit, sandwiches, etc.

If food is dished onto plates in the kitchen, participants should be encouraged to pick up and carry their plates to their table if possible. Again, independence should be encouraged.

To avoid dessert being eaten first — or the only item eaten that day — it should be held for serving until the main course has been eaten. Substitutions for participants who are diabetic should be creative and prepared in advance so they can be served along with everyone else. Red dots distinguishing diabetics should be placed on the name tags, charts, and on a list in the kitchen.

If any extra meals remain, they may be served to any participant wanting seconds. Health regulations will not allow participants to carry food home. Unused meals may be packaged, dated, and frozen for up to two weeks at the center.

Closing the Center (Appendix B5)

At the end of the day, the staff person responsible for closing the center must be certain all participants have signed out and record the time they left so that proper billing can be made at the end of the month. It is a policy that a staff person remain at the center until all clients have been picked up and/or transported home.

Before closing the center, all areas need to be straightened and cleaned for the next morning. The refrigerator should be emptied of any food that would spoil overnight (see Appendix D1.8).

The daily sign-in sheet for participants and volunteers should be checked, completed, and placed on the secretary's desk. The next day's sign-in sheet should be prepared and displayed for the staff member who opens the center the next morning.

A routine for each center should involve locking the files, desks, safe, windows, offices, and doors. Lights should be turned off and the thermostat adjusted to save on utilities.

OPERATIONAL PROCEDURES (Appendix C)

Incident Reports (Appendix C1, 2, 3)

Incident reports have been designed for a systematic method of reporting an incident. The reports assist the insurance company with documentation and provides a record of incidents to analyze and develop safeguards among all programs of the Foundation for Senior Living. Both a long and short form have been developed. The long form (Appendix C3) is used for serious incidents and the short form (Appendix C2) for minor incidents. Incident reports are sent to the corporate office at the end of each week.

Incident updates and guidelines were developed by a committee at the corporate office and have been helpful in reducing the number of serious incidents. It has also enabled the corporation to obtain lower insurance premiums.

Emergency Procedures (Appendix C4, 5)

Emergency procedures are essential for each adult day care program and must be posted by each telephone. Procedural instructions must be printed so that they can be easily read and followed. Emergencies occur regularly in adult day care programs due to the frail nature of the population being served. It is imperative that each staff member be able to respond in a quick, professional manner and that all staff be trained in basic emergency procedures, cardiopulmonary resuscitation (CPR), and the Heimlich maneuver. Emergency procedures must include instructions for calling paramedics as well as other significant persons (Appendix C5).

Unexplained Participant Absences (Appendix C6)

It is the responsibility of each client or his/her family to notify the center if they are going to be absent on their scheduled day. If an adult day care participant does not arrive at the center the day they are scheduled, and there is no notation on the sign-in sheet explaining their absence, the participant must be located to confirm that they are all right. This should be done no later than 11:00 a.m.

The participant should be called; if no answer, the emergency number listed in his/her file should be called. The transportation person (i.e., the center van driver, dial-a-ride, etc.) should be consulted. If the person cannot be located, a home visit is necessary to assess the situation. If no response at participant's residence, and after checking with neighbors, the police may need to be called for assistance.

In deciding the best action to take, personal judgment must be relied upon. Past attendance patterns will provide a clue. Above all, staff should never assume that everything is all right. It is better to be overly cautious. Staff must make sure that each participant understands the necessity of letting the center know if they will not be attending on any given day. Most often participants and their families are good about notifying the center. When an absence occurs unexpectedly, and the client cannot be located, it must be taken seriously.

Fire Drills (Appendix C7)

Fire drills are required at least every three months, but to prevent participants and staff from forgetting how to make an orderly exit from the premises, monthly fire drills should be a priority. Staff assignments for specific tasks need to be made long before a fire drill or emergency occurs. Extra wheelchairs are to be kept at each center for those who have extreme difficulty in walking.

Fire drills assist participants and staff to act responsibly should an actual emergency situation arise. It gives staff confidence that they are able to move frail elderly people out of a building in less than three minutes in a calm and organized manner.

After everyone has been taken outside, there must always be a head count of participants, staff, and volunteers to assure everyone is out of the building. This can be done by checking against the daily sign-in sheet (assignment for picking up sign-in sheet previously designated to a specific staff member).

New Participant Orientation (Appendix C8)

Each new participant in adult day care must be treated as an individual and respected for the life they held before becoming frail and in need of adult day care. Before beginning the program, the staff should meet together and learn something about the participant from the adult day care social worker who has made a home visit, written a social history, and obtained a medical form that has been filled out by the individual's physician. A plan of care can then be developed during the initial staffing using input from all staff.

A participant's first day can be traumatic. He/she may feel hesitant, frightened, angry, etc., and must be treated very gently. The social worker (see section on social services) who made the initial home visit should be on hand to greet the person when they walk in the door. The social worker should introduce the new client to the other participants and explain the day's activities. A name tag should be made after asking the new participant what he/she would like to be called. A volunteer or special participant should be asked to spend the first day with the new client. It usually takes about two days for a new participant to feel at home in the adult day care

program. Often, new participants will quickly meet other participants and develop a special friendship.

Participant Deaths/Bereavement (Appendix C9)

When a participant dies, it is important to help the surviving participants and staff express their feelings and cope with their loss. It
is not uncommon for participants who have attended the program
for years to have established a very special relationship with the
staff and other participants; a death then becomes something very
personal for those involved. An opportunity to attend the funeral
should be provided whenever possible to staff and participants.
Some participants are reassured to know that when they die, people
will care and those close to them will attend their funeral.

After a participant has died, a sympathy card signed by staff and
participants should be sent to the family. Furthermore, a discussion
should take place among the staff about the circumstances surrounding the death. Staff should be given the freedom to express
their feelings. Afterward, the participants should be brought together as a group and a picture of the deceased person may be
passed around. A discussion about the deceased participant enables
participants and staff to share special moments they had with the
person and is appropriate and often comforting.

Inquiries About Adult Day Care (Appendix C10)

When a person calls inquiring about adult day care, the call
should be channeled to the social worker, director, or nurse. They
will be able to explain the concept of adult day care, the population
being served, activities offered, and the fee. Detailed information
about funding, budgets, operation, etc., are referred to the corporate office.

When a person makes an inquiry about the center, they are referred to one of the professional staff members who can give a
professional explanation and promote the merits of the program.
Often, the paraprofessional staff sees the program from a perspective in which they are most involved (i.e., activities, meals, etc.)
and may not fully describe the total scope of the program. In addition, fee structures are best handled by a professional staff member.

Staff Communication Book (Appendix C11)

The purpose of the staff communication book is to improve communication between staff, volunteers, and participants at the adult day care center. Each staff person is responsible for reading the book every day. Each entry in the book must be signed and dated. Anything that needs to be communicated and anything that happens out of the ordinary must be written in the book.

Donations (Appendix C12)

Donations in cash and property are always needed and are welcome at each adult day care center. When a donation is made, the donor's name, address, and the amount/value of the donation are written in the communication book. Checks are made payable to the Foundation for Senior Living because the corporation has the nonprofit 501(c)(3) status. Donations can be restricted for specific programs or purposes.

It is extremely important to thank the person giving the donation verbally, and then follow with a thank-you letter signed by the program director. For large donations, the corporate office at FSL needs to be notified, and an additional thank-you letter will be sent and signed by the president/chief executive officer.

Ordering Meals and Supplies (Appendix C13)

In order to let the catering company know how many meals to plan, meals must be ordered from the caterer the Friday before the week they are needed. An estimate of the number of meals needed will be obtained by the number of participants enrolled for each of the days during the week. A standard absentee rate of 10% seems to occur in adult day care. It is important not to order too many meals because, consumed or not, the center must pay for the number of meals ordered. A "Food and Supplies Order Form" is used when ordering catered meals.

When purchasing supplies, a system that helps keep costs within the budget allocation and maximize the purchasing power of the corporation should be implemented. Small items may be purchased using petty cash and regular inventory items may be ordered from regular suppliers. These should be recorded on the "Food and Supplies Order Form." Large items are ordered through the corporate purchasing department. The system outlined in Appendix C13.1 is used. In addition, three bids for any item over $300 must be obtained. The central purchasing department handles the purchasing and obtains the bids for each individual adult day care center.

CLEANING ROUTINES (Appendix D)

In order to maintain a high standard of cleanliness and to comply with health regulations, a cleaning schedule should be implemented at each adult day care center. Daily, weekly, and monthly cleaning schedules should be followed and recorded on the cleaning checklist form.

Daily cleaning routines on items that are used routinely such as the range/oven, tables, chairs, drinking fountains, sinks, etc., should be implemented. The refrigerator should also be cleaned and unusable foods removed. Weekly cleaning schedules for ovens and monthly cleaning schedules for dry food storage areas along with defrosting the refrigerator should be implemented (see Appendix D1 for specific cleaning routines).

BOOKKEEPING PROCEDURES (Appendix E)

It is necessary to standardize bookkeeping procedures throughout the adult day care centers. Standardized procedures assist the center in maintaining good accounting principles, reduce the expense of annual audits, permit monthly reporting that enables comparisons between centers, and reduce the chance of bookkeeping errors.

Receipts (Appendix E1)

Receipts are made out on *all* monies received. All receipts must include the date, the person's name, where the money was received from; what the purpose of the transaction was (fee, donation, etc.); the amount of the transaction; a notation if it is designated for a specific purpose (scholarship, activities, etc.); and if it was to pay a fee, the amount owed, and the balance.

In order to avoid future problems, the receipt must be made in triplicate with a copy given to the person making the transaction, a copy retained at the center, and a copy sent to the corporate office. All checks should be stamped immediately with the corporate for-deposit-only bank stamp to avoid anyone taking the check and cashing it. All checks and money should be placed immediately into a cashbox (with lock) and further secured in a cabinet or safe which also can be locked.

Client Donations (Appendix E2)

Client donations are funds that are contributed by participants who do not pay a fee (see also section on Client Fees below). All other donations are considered contributions and should be designated as such when writing a receipt or making a deposit. It is important to separate the incoming revenue into categories in order to keep track of the fund-raising efforts being made, the community support, and the client fees and donations to the program.

In order to maximize the amount of dollars being donated by the clients, the following system has been developed. Each morning before the participants arrive, a donation envelope is attached to the participant's name badge. This will be a daily reminder to donate what they can to the program. In many instances, participants' self-esteem and independence are strengthened when they are able to donate. The envelope system provides an opportunity to donate without feeling pressured to give beyond their means.

Discretion is the key to a successful donation program. Letters to the family regarding the need for donations should be sent out periodically. Some families will choose to donate monthly, others weekly. An individualized system for all clients who are not paying the full fee is worth the time spent.

Deposits (Appendix E3)

Deposits must be made in a timely manner, once or twice a week, depending on the amount of incoming dollars. Cash flow is very important for any small business and it is important for this reason alone that deposits be made as timely as possible. In addition, for security reasons it is better to make frequent deposits.

Client Fees (Appendix E4)

Client fees are charged to any client for whom the center is not being reimbursed (usually by government funds) for his/her care. The fee is based on the number of hours they are at the center. There is an hourly fee with a minimum of four hours per day and not less than two days per week. Each participant must have a plan of care and an opportunity to work toward their goals at least eight hours each week.

Monthly billing statements are sent to the client or his/her family. Many times, his/her family will choose to pay the bill for the family member, and they do not want the fee or bill discussed with the family member. Again, discretion must be used.

Spread Sheets (Appendix E5)

Spread sheets are used to post the daily hours each participant attends the center to collect statistics, fill out required reports, and bill the fee-paying clients for the service. It is necessary to post these hours of service each day to eliminate the cumbersome task at the end of each month. These sheets must be proofread and the director of the program must sign them at the end of each month, acknowledging that they were proofread and are accurate.

Petty Cash (Appendix E6)

Petty cash is used for small purchases that are not ordered from a vendor. Petty cash documentation is essential and each purchase must have a receipt designating what the purchase is and what line item in the budget is to be charged (arts and crafts, food, etc.). A limited number of people on the staff should have access to the petty cash funds, and funds should be locked in a file or safe at all times.

SOCIAL SERVICES (Appendix F)

Social services are an integral component of each adult day care program. Social services are provided by a professional social worker who has a degree in social work and/or counseling. The social services provided in an adult day care center include individual and family counseling, crisis intervention, accessing clients to needed services in the community, assisting clients with alternative living arrangements, leading group discussions, holding meetings for the families of the participants, providing all client intake services and assessments, and facilitating the marketing function of the program in locating clients who are able to pay the full fee of the service.

Client Intake (Appendix F2)

Before a new participant is admitted to the program, the social worker makes a home visit to the client's home. This is done to gain a better understanding of the environment in which the participant lives. This time provides an excellent opportunity to assess the client's orientation, ability to perform daily living skills, and to determine just how the person is managing in his/her environment. A social history is a narrative written about the client that tells the reason for referral, a physical description of the client's present situation, and some general impressions and recommendations about the person. A social history is the key to developing an initial plan of care for the client. This care plan is completed before the client ever begins the program.

In addition, the social worker obtains a medical form completed by the client's physician, completes a social (Appendix F3) and physical (Appendix F4) assessment, and provides the family with information about fees, transportation, and the program in general. After all the information has been gathered and a plan of care is completed, the social worker will set up the schedule with the adult day care participant and they will begin the program.

Participant Care Plans (Appendix F6)

Each client must have an individual care plan (i.e., staffing, individual program plan) that is developed by the adult day care staff using an interdisciplinary team approach. Family and client input is vital to developing a care plan. Client care plans enable the staff to provide a coordinated effort to help the individual achieve his/her goals.

Participants have an initial care plan that is developed before they begin the adult day care program. A follow-up plan is developed two weeks after the person begins the program. Each subsequent staffing of the individual occurs at a minimum of once every six months, but the average amount of time between clients' care plan is three months.

Progress Notes (Appendix F7)

Progress notes are written monthly on each client enrolled in the adult day care program. They are kept in the individual client's file. The purpose of monthly progress notes is to document the person's progress toward his/her goals and objectives as developed in the care plan. Progress notes also force a staff person to review each client monthly.

Progress notes are a safe check so that individuals do not get "lost" in the system. There are many clients with severe problems that require many hours of staff care. The "little ladies who crochet" may get overlooked if it were not for this system that forces one to analyze their needs each month.

Narratives (Appendix F8)

Narratives are written on each individual every six months and upon discharge from the program. They are written by the social worker and retained in the client's file. The purpose of a narrative is to add anything to the file that might increase the knowledge and understanding by the other staff about the client. A closing narrative is written when a person leaves the program. This provides a way to track the client and record information that may be needed in the future for statistical purposes.

HEALTH SURVEILLANCE (Appendix G)

Adult day care centers cater to the frail elderly who have a myriad of health problems. The health condition of frail elderly clients is poor and they suffer from chronic conditions that accentuate their frailty. The majority of health problems are heart, circulatory, and diabetes-related.

It is necessary that the health status of each client is monitored closely, while encouraging independence, rehabilitation, and restoration (NIAD/NCOA). This "wellness" approach promotes independence and discourages participants from taking on a "sick" role. An overdependency on health care can lead to a decline in the ability to function independently. Therefore, the frail clients are given the opportunity to achieve the highest level of independence possible, while at the same time they are monitored closely so that their health does not deteriorate. When a deterioration in health does occur, it becomes imperative that the staff at the center recognize the change and immediately report it to the center nurse so he/she can provide the appropriate intervention.

All adult day care programs operated by the Foundation for Senior Living employ registered nurses. The center nurse must work independently, be confident in his/her decisions, and possess the ability to work closely with each individual's physician. Center nurses are asked to wear street clothes instead of nurse's uniforms in order to promote a "wellness model" of health care. Community health nurses usually do very well in an adult day care center environment, and they seem to feel more comfortable in this style of nursing than do nurses who are accustomed to working in hospitals.

Health Monitoring (Appendix G1)

Health monitoring of an individual's blood pressure, pulse, and weight is performed at a minimum of once a month. In most cases these services are performed more often by the center nurse. Staff, volunteers, and participants are encouraged to report immediately any change in a client's behavior/condition to the center nurse who, in turn, will assess the client's needs and intervene whenever necessary.

ACTIVITIES (Appendix H)

Each adult day care center's activity program is different and takes into account each participant's individuality and its staff's creativity. Though certain activities are basic to every adult day care program, the scope and variety of the activities are largely determined by the participants' needs, abilities, and interests. Every day should, however, be structured and purposeful.

The purpose of each adult day care center's activity program is to provide therapeutic and rehabilitative activities for its participants. An awareness of the frailty of the elderly and their functional limitations and abilities is important for the staff and the volunteers to understand when developing an activities program. Major considerations when planning an activities program include the balance of participant and staff involvement, the high energy activities which are offered in the earlier part of the day when energy levels are highest, the importance of alternating high energy activities with quiet time activities, and the provision of equal spacing of time between meals and snacks.

VOLUNTEERS (Appendix I)

Volunteers are vital to provide top quality care to participants in an adult day care center. Since volunteers bring an added dimension to the program, each volunteer must feel needed, wanted, purposeful, and appreciated. Volunteers must be given the training and guidelines just like the staff and allowed to give input into the program. Some programs fall into a bad habit of expecting the volunteers to do all the routine, mundane chores that the staff does not like to do. This must never happen!

There must be good rapport between paid staff and the volunteers. Volunteers are not a replacement for staff. Each volunteer and staff member must understand the differences in responsibilities between volunteer and staff positions. Volunteers must be given proper encouragement, praise, and feedback in order to maintain their enthusiasm for the vastly needed work they perform at the center. Volunteers can be the center's best spokesmen. If volunteers are happy, know they are appreciated, and truly understand the purpose of the adult day care program, they will virtually tell the world. One could not buy better advertising!

PERSONAL HYGIENE (Appendix J)

Older people, like all other people, have individualized ways of taking care of their personal hygiene. Some people are meticulous, others are not. The frail elderly may have suffered from a number of losses that can hinder their ability to totally maintain their personal hygiene. Adult day care staff must be helpful to individuals experiencing poor personal hygiene by assisting them in obtaining additional home services if needed, and by teaching them how to maintain their personal hygiene so they are socially acceptable.

Bathroom Accidents (Appendix J1)

Bathroom accidents are likely to occur among adult day care participants because of their limited mobility, not necessarily because they are incontinent. Their ability to hurry is often impeded and even with proper planning an occasional bathroom accident occurs. When a participant has a bathroom accident, the situation must be handled with tact and with the least possible embarrassment. Depending on the situation, the participant will probably need assistance, and most often the family will need to be notified because the person may be sick or need a change of clothes.

MONTHLY REPORTS (Appendix K)

There are a variety of reports and forms that need to be completed on a monthly basis in order to document the care that was provided for billing purposes, government contracts, and statistics. Samples of some of the monthly report forms can be found in Appendix K.

SUMMARY

America is a nation that is aging. During recent decades recognizable advances in the health care industry and the apparent success in refinements of care have increased demands for service. In view of these convergent and growing needs for innovative approaches to treatment/care for the elderly, a relatively new concept has found its place among the long-term care services. Adult day

care is a program designed to assist frail elderly and physically impaired adults by providing health surveillance, personal care, supervision, and an organized program of activities and therapies in a
protective setting.

Adult day care centers have made a tremendous impact over the
past 15 years. They offer several advantages that are distinct from
other long-term care services. The uniqueness of adult day care
allows the participants to continue living in their community, relieves the family of total 24-hour care, and is cost-effective. Adult
day care is responsive to the demand for quality care at an acceptable cost. As a result, adult day care centers exist throughout the
nation and are providing a valuable service in each community in
which they are located.

References

Arizona Statewide Health Coordinating Council and the Arizona Department of Health Services Bureau of Health, Economic and Planning Series (1982). *Arizona State Health Plan 1982-1987*. Phoenix, AZ: Arizona Department of Health Series.

Barnes, J. (1974). The effects of reality orientation classroom in memory loss, comprehension, and disorientation in geriatric patients. *The Gerontologist, 14,* 138-142.

Benedek, T. (1970). Parenthood during the life cycle. In E.J. Anthony (Ed.), *Parenthood* (p. 20). Boston: Little, Brown & Co.

Bourque, P. (1984, April). Deputy Administrator, Health Care Financing Administration. Speech, Washington, DC.

Brickel, C.M. (1979). The therapeutic roles of cat mascots with a hospital-based geriatric population: A staff survey. *Gerontologist, 19,* 368-372.

Brody, S.J. (1980). The graying of America. *Hospitals, 54,* 65.

Brook, P., Degun, G. & Mather, M. (1975). Reality orientation: A therapy for psychogeriatric patients. *British Journal of Psychiatry, 127,* 42-45.

Butler, R.N. (1974). Successful aging and the role of the life-review. *Journal of the American Geriatric Society, 22,* 529-535.

Butler, R. & Lewis, M. (1973). *Aging and mental health positive psychosocial approaches*. St. Louis: C.V. Mosby.

Butler, R.N. (1963). The life review: An interpretation of reminiscence in the aged. *Psychiatry, 26,* 65-75.

Butler, R.N. & Lewis, M. (1982). *Aging and mental health: A positive psychological and biomedical approach* (3rd ed.). St. Louis: C.V. Mosby.

Carter, M.J., Van Andel, G.E. & Robb, G.M. (1985). *Therapeutic recreation: A practical guide*. St. Louis: Times Mirror/Mosby College Publication.

Citrin, R.S. & Dixon, D.N. (1977). Reality orientation: A milieu therapy used in an institution for the aged. *The Gerontologist, 17,* 39-43.

Corbin, S.J. (1980). Games of rapport. *Canadian Counsellor, 14*(2), 99-101.

Corbin, S. & Nelson, T.M. (1980). Using angels and devils: A board game developed for play in nursing homes. *International Journal of Aging and Human Development, 11*(3), 243-250.

Corson, S.A., Corson, E.O & Dehass, D. et al. (1976). The socializing role of pet animals in nursing homes: An experiment in nonverbal communication therapy. In *Proceedings from the International Symposium on Society Stress and Disease: Aging and Old Age*.

Cosin, L. (1971, June 15). Presentation of the philosophy and practice of total patient care. Hearings before the Subcommittee on Long-Term Care, Special Committee on Aging, U.S. Senate, Part 14.

Cosin, L.Z., Mort, M., Post, F., Westropp, C. & Williams, M. (1958, April). Experimental treatment of persistent senile confusion. *The International Journal of Social Psychiatry*, *4*(2), 24-42.

Department of Economic Security (1977). *Certification standards for adult day-care*.

Dolan, M.B. (1980). Day-care for the elderly. In I. Burnside (Ed.), *Psychosocial nursing care of the aged*. New York: McGraw-Hill.

Dunton, W.R. & Licht, S. (1950). *Occupational therapy: Principles and practice*. Springfield, IL: Charles C Thomas.

Ebersole, P.P. (1978). Establishing reminiscing groups. In I.M. Burnside (Ed.), *Working with the elderly: Group process and techniques*. North Scituate, MA: Duxbury Press.

Ernst, M. & Shore, H. (1977). *Sensitizing people to the process-of-aging: The in-service educator's guide*. Denton: North Texas State University.

Farber, S.J. (1983). Development of geriatrics. In *Proceedings of the Regional Institutes on Geriatrics and Medical Education* (p. 29). Washington, DC: Association of American Medical Colleges.

Fersh, I.E. (1980). Dance/movement therapy: A holistic approach to working with the elderly. *Activities, Adaptation & Aging*, *1*, 21-30.

Folsom, J.C. (1966). Elderly patients found responsive to program of reality orientation. *Psychiatric Progress*, *1*, 1-3.

Folsom, J.C. (1968). Reality orientation for the elderly mental patient. *Journal of Geriatric Psychiatry*, *1*, 291-307.

Foundation for Senior Living (files) (1983). 3507 N. Central Avenue, Suite 500, Phoenix, AZ 85012.

Galton, L. (1979). *The truth about senility and how to avoid it*. New York: Thomas & Crowell.

Golightly, E.K., Bossenmaier, M.M., McChesney, J.A., Williams, B.S. & Wyble, S.J. (1984, May). Planning to meet the needs of the hospitalized elderly. *The Journal of Nursing Administration*, 29-39.

Gotestam, K. (1980). Behavior and dynamic psychotherapy with the elderly. In J.E. Birren & R.B. Sloane (Eds.), *Handbook of mental health and aging*. Englewood Cliffs, NJ: Prentice Hall.

Green, I. (1975). *Housing for the elderly*. New York: Van Nostrand Reinhold Co.

Hanley, I.G., McGuire, E.J. & Byrd, W.D. (1981). Reality orientation and dementia: A controlled study of two approaches. *British Journal of Psychiatry*, *138*, 10-14.

Hasselkus, B.R. & Kiernat, J.M. (1973). Independent living for the elderly. *American Journal of Occupational Therapy*, *27*, 181-188.

Health Care Financing Administration (1980). *Directory of adult day-care centers*. Washington, DC: HCFA, DHHS.

Hickey, T. (1974). In-service training in gerontology. *The Gerontologist, 14*(1), 57-64.

Kahana, B. & Kahana, E. (1970). Grandparenthood from the perspective of the developing grandchild. *Developmental Psychology, 3*, 98-105.

Kartman, L.L. (1980, Fall). The power of music with patients in a nursing home. *Activities, Adaptation & Aging, 1*(1), 9-17.

Kraus, R. (1978). *Therapeutic recreation service: Principles and practices*. Philadelphia: W.B. Saunders Company.

Langdon, H.J. & Langdon, L.L. (1983). *Initiating occupational therapy programs within the public school system: A guide for occupational therapists and public school administrators*. Thorofare, NJ: Slack, Inc.

Leonard, L. (1978). *Counseling the elderly: Adult day-care*. New York: Springer.

Levinson, B.M. (1972). *Pets and human development*. Springfield, IL: Charles C Thomas.

Levinson, B.M. (1978). Pets and personality development. *Psychological Reports, 42*, 1031-1038.

Lewis, M.I. & Butler, R.N. (1974). Life review therapy: Putting memories to work in individual and group psychotherapy. *Geriatrics, 29*, 165-173.

LoGerfo, M. (1980). Three ways of reminiscence in theory and practice. *International Journal of Aging and Human Development, 12*, 39-48.

Lorronde, S. (1983). Adopt-a-grandparent. *Modern Maturity, 26*, 50, 52.

MacDonald, E.M. (1964). *Occupational therapy in rehabilitation*. Baltimore, MD: The Williams and Wilkins Company.

McCuan, E.R. (1973). An evaluation of a geriatric day-care center as a parallel service to institutional care. Project of the Levindale Geriatric Research Center, Baltimore, MD.

McMahon, A.W. & Rhudick, P.J. (1964). Reminiscing adaptational significance in the aged. *Archives of General Psychiatry, 10*, 292-298.

Meyerhoff, B.C. & Tufte, V. (1975). Life history as integration: An essay on an experimental model. *The Gerontologist, 15*, 541-543.

Middleton, L. (1984). *Alzheimer's family support groups: A manual for group facilitators*. Tampa, FL: Suncoast Gerontology Center, U.S.F. Medical Center.

Mitchell, R.A. (1966). Reality orientation for brain damaged patients. *Staff Magazine, 3*(3), 3-4.

Molinari, V. & Reichlin, R.E. (1984-1985). Life review reminiscence in the elderly: A review of the literature. *International Journal of Aging and Human Development, 20*(2), 81-92.

Mugford, R.A. & M'Comiskey, J.G. (1975). Some work on the psychotherapeutic value of caged birds with old people. In R.S. Anderson (Ed.), *Pets, animals, and society*. London: Bailler Tindall.

National Institute of Adult Day-Care (1984, April). *National standards*. Washington, DC: National Council on Aging.

Nystrom, E.P. (1974). Activity patterns and leisure concepts among the elderly. *American Journal of Occupational Therapy, 28*, 337-345.

O'Brien, C. (1980). Exploring geriatric care: An alternative to institutionalization. *Geriatric Nursing*.

Oregon State University Extension Service (1983). New game helps solve dilemmas of aging. *Aging*, 39.

Padula, H. (1983). *Developing adult day-care*. Washington, DC: National Council on Aging.

Palmer, M.D. (1980, Fall). Music therapy and gerontology. *Activities, Adaptation and Aging, 1*(1), 37-40.

Pardini, A. (1984, April-May). Exercise, vitality and aging. *Aging*, 19-29.

Pincus, A. (1970). Reminiscence in aging and its implications for social work practice. *Social Work, 15*, 47-53.

Pritzlaff Commission on Long-Term Care (1984, July). *Long-Term Care in Arizona* (Executive Summary). Phoenix, AZ: Flynn Foundation.

Robb, S.S. & Stegman, C.E. (1983). Companion animals and elderly people: A challenge for evaluators of social support. *The Gerontologist, 23*(3), 277-282.

Roos, N.J., Shapiro, E. & Roos, L.L. (1984). Aging and the demand for health services: Which aged and whose demand? *The Gerontologist, 24*(1), 31-36.

Sandel, S.L. (1978). Reminiscence in movement therapy with the aged. *Art Psychotherapy, 5*, 217-221.

Silden, I. (1983). In a warm puppy, a new lease on life. *Modern Maturity, 28*(1), 72, 74-76.

Snider, L. (1976). *Working paper: An analysis of adult day-care in the United States*. Unpublished paper. Boston: Boston University Gerontology Center.

Solomon, K. (1982). Social antecedents of learned helplessness in the health care setting. *The Gerontologist, 22*, 282-287.

Spear, M. (1970). *The guide for in-service training for development services for older persons: A report of the American Public Welfare Association project*. Chicago: Public Welfare Project on Aging.

Taulbee, L. & Folsom, J.C. (1966). Reality orientation for geriatric patients. *Hospital Community Psychiatry, 17*, 23-25.

U.S. Bureau of the Census (1983). *America in transition: An aging society*. Washington, DC: U.S. Government Printing Office.

U.S. Department of Commerce. Bureau of the Census (1983). *1980 census of the population. Vol. I: Characteristics of the population in Chapter B: General population on characteristics Part IV-S. Summary series PC80-1B1*. Washington, DC: U.S. Government Printing Office.

U.S. Department of Health and Human Services (1980). *Vital and health statistics*. Washington, DC: Public Health Service, National Center for Health Statistics.

University of Michigan (1981). *Audiovisual aids for the environment*. Michigan: Institute of Gerontology.

Warren, H.H. (1977). Self-perception of independence among urban elderly. *American Journal of Occupational Therapy, 31*, 71-74.

Weisman, S. (1983). Computer games for the frail elderly. *The Gerontologist, 23*(4), 361-363.

Weisman, S. (1983). Nursing home residents savor a new kind of "apple." *Aging, 337*, 29-30.

Weiss, J.C. (1979). *The use of art and writing as therapeutic tools for improving reality orientation for OBS or brain dysfunction patients*. Unpublished master's thesis. Lone Mountain College.

Weiss, J.C. (1980). The use of art and writing as therapeutic tools for improving reality orientation. *Activities, Adaptation & Aging, 1*, 3-8.

Wilson, C.C. & Netting, F.E. (1983). Companion animals and the elderly: A state-of-the-art summary. *The Journal of the American Veterinary Medical Association, 183*(12), 1425-1429.

Wood, V. (1982). Grandparenthood: An ambiguous role. *Generations, VII*(2), 22-23, 35.

Woods, R.T. (1979). Reality orientation and staff attention: A controlled study. *British Journal of Psychiatry, 134*, 502-507.

Zeiger, B.L. (1976). Life review in art therapy with the aged. *American Journal of Art Therapy, 15*, 47-50.

APPENDIXES

FSL Adult Day Care Operations Manual

The following represents a model of an operations/procedures manual. It is not to be taken as a document to use when beginning the operations of an adult day care center. It should, however, be used as an example of some of the areas one should include when developing a manual.

A. *Adult Day Care Statement of Purpose*

Adult day care is a community-based service that assists frail elderly people and physically handicapped adults to remain living in their own homes, with their family, or in a sheltered living situation for as long as possible. Independence is the goal for each adult day care participant. Each individual's remaining abilities are enhanced so that he or she can become as independent as possible.

An adult day care center provides a gamut of health and social services in a congregate setting. A variety of programs including a nursing component, recreation, activities of daily living, counseling, nutrition, transportation, and rehabilitation are all offered in adult day care.

Most adult day care clients fall into the category of being *disabled*, *depressed*, or *disoriented* to the degree that they are unable to function in any other type of program, yet 24-hour nursing care is not required.

Adult day care offers an individualized plan of care to meet the needs of each participant. Adult day care assists families and spouses of disabled persons provides a safe and stimulating environment for their family member while they are at work. It also helps to increase the independence of a participant who may have suffered a stroke or may have become disabled. For the participant experiencing disorientation, adult day care assists that person in relearning basic daily living skills and provides daily reality orientation.

Adult day care provides an excellent opportunity for a frail elderly or disabled person to remain living in the community at a relatively low cost. The cost of most adult day care programs average $15.00 to $20.00 per day. Many adult day care centers use Social Service Block Grant Funds, Title III, United Way, scholarship funds, and private donations to assist participants in the payment for the service.

Adult day care is an exciting alternative in the delivery of long-term care services that has produced dynamic results for participants and their families.

B. *Routine Daily Procedures*

B1 — Opening the Center

1. Unlock all doors, open drapes and windows if desired, turn on lights, adjust thermostat, unlock file cabinets and desk drawers.
2. Place contribution envelopes out.
3. Place correct daily participant sign-in/sign-out sheet in assigned area, along with the name tags for participants scheduled to attend that day.
4. Review snack menu for the day. Check for participants on special diets and arrange correct substitutions.
5. Check monthly schedule for special events. If a special event is scheduled for that day, make necessary preparations.
6. Check schedule to see if any center visitors are scheduled.
7. Check volunteer schedule. If volunteers are scheduled

for that day, have name tags prepared and job assignments ready.

8. Put *Staff Communication Book* in assigned place.
9. Make coffee for the day. Place cups, creamers, sugar, and stirrers in serving area.
10. Make sure that the *Nutritional Supplementation Daily Participation Sign-In/Sign-Out Sheet* is correctly prepared and placed in the assigned location.
11. Check to see that bathrooms have enough paper products and soap.

B2 — Greeting Routine

1. Meet the van or transportation vehicle and assist the driver in unloading the participants.
2. As the participants enter the center, greet them *warmly*, and help them to hang up their coats (if assistance is needed).
3. Have the participants sign their names and time (if coming by private car) on the *Participant Sign-In/Sign-Out Sheet*. Be sure they sign in both places. Assist if necessary.
4. Have them put on their name tags.
5. Offer some coffee and show them where it is kept. If possible, have the participant prepare and carry their own coffee to the table.
6. Record any pertinent information regarding the participants' condition in the staff communication book.
7. If absences are phoned in, record this on the *Participant Sign-In/Sign-Out Sheet*.

B3 — Snack Procedure

(Allow about 1/2 hour for snack preparation)

1. Be sure and wash hands before handling food.
2. Be sure that people on special diets have substitutions planned.
3. As much as possible, have people serve themselves and help others who can't.

4. After snack, let participants carry their own plates, glasses, etc., back to kitchen.
5. Wash dishes using method outlined in Dishwashing Procedures.

Some notes . . . .
a. Encourage independence and self-sufficient behavior.
b. Offer a variety of snacks; use your imagination!

B4 — Lunch Procedure

1. Allow approximately 1/2 hour for lunch preparation if using catered meals. Longer if preparing meals.
2. Have participants wipe tables using 1/2 capful of bleach in one gallon water solution.
3. Have participants set the tables:
   a. Placemat.
   b. Glass for milk/coffee cup.
   c. Fork, knife, spoon.
   d. Salt, pepper.
   e. Napkin.
   f. Plate (if food is dished out at table).
4. Staff must wash hands before serving food and encourage participants to wash their hands before eating.
5. Place food attractively on plates.
6. If food is dished on plates in the kitchen, encourage participants to come and get their plates and carry them to the table if possible.
7. Encourage pleasant mealtime conversation.
8. Talk about the meal; how it's prepared, etc.
9. Serve dessert after the main meal.
10. Have participants carry their own plates back to the kitchen. *Encourage independence.*
11. After lunch, have the participants sign the *Nutritional Supplementation Sheet.*
12. Have participant wipe the table with disinfectant solution.

NOTE: If any extra meals remain after everyone has been served lunch, freeze the meal and write the date and contents on the cover. Meals can be frozen for a maximum of two weeks.

B5 – Closing the Center

1. *Do not, under any circumstances,* leave a participant alone at the Center!! DO NOT LEAVE until all participants have been picked up.
2. Look at all areas to be sure they have been cleaned.
3. Go through the refrigerator and check that all foodstuffs are properly labeled and dated. Discard any food that won't remain fresh overnight.
4. Review *Participant Sign-In/Sign-Out Sheet* and *Nutritional Supplementation Daily Participant Sign-In/Sign-Out Sheet*. Make sure they are completed and accurate.
5. Check *Volunteer Registration* to be sure all volunteer time has been recorded.
6. Return furniture to original placement (if specified in lease agreement).
7. Lock all participant files.
8. Lock all file drawers, desk drawers, safe, and cabinets.
9. Lock all doors and windows, pull drapes, turn off lights, adjust thermostat, make sure outside bathrooms are locked and the lights turned off.

C. *Operational Procedures*

C1 – Incident Reports

1. Use long form if incident is serious:
   a. Participant is injured.
   b. Staff is injured.
   c. Volunteer is injured.
   d. When a paramedic is called.
   e. Serious illness.
   f. Property loss (of any significant value).
   g. Wandering by participant.

NOTE: In addition to long form, note incident on weekly form sent to FSL.

2. Note incident on short form if incident is minor:
An event that happens often (i.e., participant locks self
in bathroom, no injuries involved).

NOTE: If in doubt, use long form.

3. Follow time periods set by FSL for reporting Emergency Incidents.

C2 - Incident Report Form

FOUNDATION FOR SENIOR LIVING

FACILITY, PROGRAM OR PRODUCT_____ DATE_____

TO: Field Director_____ (Name)

INCIDENT REPORT

Routing:

Incident report should be filled out by staff member involved in, or
witnessing the incident. Report then should be passed to immediate supervisor who reviews and forwards to his corporate supervisors.

Date of Incident_____ Time_____A.M./P.M.

Location of Incident_____

Nature of Incident_____

Employee who is filling out incident report:

Name_____ Title_____

Phone Number_____

Person(s) involved:

Client: Name_____ Phone_____

         Address_____

Apparent status of client before incident:

               Physical   Mental

Good_____ Fair_____   Completely oriented_____
Poor_____   Appeared confused _____

Description of incident: (Include circumstances under which incident
occurred.)

_____

_____

_____

Remarks: (Client, family, witnesses, etc.)_____
_____
_____

Witnesses, if any:

Name_____ Phone_____

Address_____

Name_____ Phone_____

Address_____

Extent and Character of injury and part(s) of body affected:

_____

_____

Were paramedics called?   Yes___ No___

Was a physician called?   Yes___ No___

Treatment, if any:_____

_____

Suggestion(s) on how to prevent similar incidents:_____

_____

_____

Final disposition (what was the outcome?)_____

_____

_____

Immediate supervisor's comments: _____

_____

                              _____   _____
                                   signature   date

Home Care, Maricopa: Was it reported to case management? Yes___ No___

Comments:_____ Date_____

Corporate supervisor's comments: _____

_____

                              _____   _____
                                   signature   date

FACILITY, PROGRAM OR PROJECT _____   WEEK ENDING _____

BY _____

Date	Time	Location	Name	Nature of Incident and Disposition

C3 – Incident Report Log

94

C4 - Emergency Incidents

MEMORANDUM FOR THE RECORD: JANUARY 5, 1983

TO: ALL PERSONNEL
FROM: INCIDENT PREVENTION COUNCIL
SUBJECT: EMERGENCY INCIDENTS

FOR YOUR GUIDANCE, THE FOLLOWING MINIMUM TIME PERIODS ARE TO BE OBSERVED
FOR THE REPORTING OF INCIDENTS. YOUR SUPERVISOR AND/OR A MEMBER OF THE
CORPORATE STAFF MUST BE CONTACTED WITHIN THE TIME INDICATED:

SERIOUS INJURY   IMMEDIATELY

DEATH - UNUSUAL CIRCUMSTANCES   IMMEDIATELY

DEATH - NORMAL CIRCUMSTANCES   NEXT DAY

CLIENT/PATIENT MISSING   ½ HOUR

SERIOUS DAMAGE TO PREMISES   1 HOUR

AN INCIDENT PREVENTION CARD LISTING THE TELEPHONE NUMBERS OF ALL INCIDENT
PREVENTION COUNCIL MEMBERS HAS BEEN PROVIDED TO ALL SUPERVISORY STAFF.

C5 — Emergency Procedures

Procedure to Follow in Case of Medical Emergency

1. DO NOT PANIC ! ! !
2. Evaluate the situation.
3. Call the paramedics.
4. Speak clearly.
5. State nature of problem.
6. Give correct address of the center.
7. Get the participant's case file.
8. Contact participant's family.

9. Have a staff member remain with the participant at all times.

C6 — Unexplained Absence Follow-up

If an ADC participant does not arrive at the center by 11:00 a.m. and there has not been an absence report filled in on the sign-in sheet or staff communication book:

1. Check with transportation to see if the absence was called in to the driver.
2. If not reported, call the participant's home phone number.
3. If no answer, call the emergency numbers listed on the participant's record.
4. If the participant lives alone, take immediate action:
   a. Send a staff member to the participant's home to assess the situation.
   b. If no response, call the police and report the situation.

NOTE: Use personal judgement in assessing the urgency of the situation. Past attendance patterns may provide a clue. Be overly sensitive to the situation rather than "assume" everything is all right.

C7 — Fire Drills

1. Fire drills must be held at least every three months.
2. During the drill, the ADC staff should act as if it were a real fire emergency.
3. The drill procedure is as follows:
   a. The director rings the fire bell.
   b. Staff members lead the participants in an orderly manner to a designated area outside away from the building.
   c. The activity coordinator is responsible for bringing the attendance sheet with her and taking roll once all participants are outside.
   d. The director is responsible for checking the facility to

make sure all participants, staff, and volunteers are outside.
e. Once all participants, staff, and volunteers are accounted for, reenter the building.

4. After the fire drill, a report is sent to the Corporate ADC Field Director. It should contain:
   a. The date and time of the drill.
   b. The number of staff, participants, and volunteers present.
   c. The amount of time it took to vacate the building.
   d. Any problems that occurred.
   e. Suggestions for improving the performance.
   f. Where the alleged "fire" occurred. (Example: in trash can by secretary's desk.)

C8 — Procedure for New Participant Orientation

1. Social worker* notifies ADC staff prior to beginning date and present at staff meeting.
2. Social worker to be on hand to be first to greet new participant.
3. Greet the participant and ask how they would like to be addressed (example: Mrs. Smith or Jane Smith).
4. Prepare a name tag:
   a. Name of participant.
   b. Name and phone number of the ADC Center.
   c. If the participant is diabetic, place a red dot on his/her name tag *and* on the outside of their file folder. Add their name to the list of diabetics in the kitchen.
5. New participants to be introduced to staff.
6. Social worker then turns new participant over to activity coordinator.
7. Activity coordinator introduces new participant to other participants.
8. Activity coordinator appoints staff member or volunteer or student or participant to act as special "buddy" for the first day.

*Director may substitute for social worker or activity coordinator.

C9 — Helping the Participants To Deal With Bereavement

When a participant dies, it is important to help the surviving participants and staff express their feelings and cope with their loss. The following points may be helpful:

1. Talk with the staff, discuss the circumstances surrounding the death and share feelings.
2. Assemble the center participants in a large group. If possible, share a picture of the deceased participant. Share feelings and encourage the participants to talk about it.
3. If possible, arrange for participants to attend the funeral services.
4. Pass around a sympathy card and have all the participants and staff sign it, then send it to the family.

NOTE: It is important to allow staff and participants to attend the funeral of a participant who has died. However, no one should be forced to do so.

C10 — Inquiries About Adult Day Care

Telephone Inquiry

1. Refer phone call to ADC director, social worker or nurse.
2. Explain what adult day care is:
   a. Type of people we serve in ADC.
   b. What hours the Center is open.
   c. What days the Center is open.
   d. Type of activities that are offered.
   e. What the fee is.
3. Do not give detailed information on funding sources, budgets, etc. If that information is desired, refer the call to FSL offices.

In-Person Inquiry

1. Get the social worker, director, or nurse.
2. Show the individuals around the ADC Center.

3. Follow the same procedure in answering questions as outlined in *telephone inquiries*.

C11 — Staff Communication Book

The purpose of the *Staff Communication Book* is to improve communications at the ADC Center. Every staff person is responsible for reading this book every day. Each entry should be signed and dated. Examples of information recorded:

1. Expected staff absences (write on the date you expect to be absent).
2. Detailed reasons for participant's absence.
3. Special messages for van drivers.

NOTE: A staff communication book can be a loose-leaf notebook with plenty of room to add to.

C12 — Donations

1. Record donor's name and address and value of donation (if applicable).
2. Express your gratitude verbally.
3. Send a Thank-You letter on FSL stationery.

C13 — Ordering Meals and Supplies

Supplies

1. Check inventory weekly, especially those items which are depleted rapidly.
2. Make a list of needed items.
3. Depending on the item:
   a. Use petty cash funds and purchase the item. OR
   b. Place order with appropriate supplier.
4. Record, using the *Food and Supplies Order Form*.
5. Use FSL Purchasing Department for large items (paper goods, office supplies, equipment, etc.).

Meals

1. Order meals on the Friday before the week they are needed.
2. Check the permanent attendance lists and estimate the number of meals needed each day:
   a. Subtract meals for participants that have reported they will not attend the ADC the following week.
   b. Add meals for new participants and staff who eat at the ADC Center.
3. Record, using the *catered meals* form.
4. Staff are allowed to purchase meals at the full cost of the meal.

D. *Cleaning Routines*

Daily	*Weekly*	*Monthly*
Electric Range	Refrigerator	Dry Food Storage
Coffee Urn	Dishwashing	Storage Room
Tables, Chairs,	Machine	Cabinets
Counters	Coffee Urn Gauge	Defrost Refrigerators
Can Opener	Ovens	Wash Walls in Kitchen,
Carts		if needed
Floors		
Sinks		

D1—Specific Cleaning Routines

Electric Range

1. Wash range daily after it has cooled; use warm water and a mild detergent to remove greasy film; rinse with clear water and dry. Take care that water does not get into the electrical elements.
2. Wipe surfaces made of iron with an oiled cloth to prevent rusting.

Coffee Urns

1. Remove urn bag as soon as coffee is made. Wash in cold water.

2. Empty urn daily, rinse thoroughly in clear, hot water; scour with a good detergent, special urn cleaner, or baking soda to remove discoloration; rinse thoroughly, first with hot water, then with cold.
3. Clean gauges with special brush.

Tables, Chairs, Counters

1. Clean daily.
2. As soon as tables have been cleared, wipe table tops and soiled surfaces with disinfectant solution (1/2 capful bleach to one gallon hot water).
3. Dry surfaces with a clean cloth.
4. Check floors for spills!

Can Opener

1. Clean daily.
2. Wipe all surfaces with disinfectant solution.
3. Check cutting edge for stickiness.
4. Dry with clean cloth.

Carts

1. Clean daily.
2. Wipe all surfaces with disinfectant solution.
3. Check for food spills and dried food.
4. Dry with clean cloth.

Floors

1. Check daily.
2. Even if the center has a janitorial service, center staff must be aware of all spilled liquid and foods. Wipe all spills immediately!
3. Keep floor free from trash.

Sinks

1. Clean daily.
2. Wipe after every use; once daily, wipe out using disinfectant solution or cleanser.

3. Use Clorox for stains.
4. Wipe surrounding surfaces.

Refrigerator

1. Check daily for unusable foodstuffs.
2. Wrap and label items that are perishable.
3. Clean thoroughly *every* week:
   a. Remove all foodstuffs.
   b. Wash shelves and walls using warm water and detergent. If necessary, scour with a stiff brush, rinse with a weak solution of baking soda or borax; dry thoroughly.
4. Defrost refrigerator *monthly*.
   a. Remove all foodstuffs.
   b. Turn temperature to *off*.
   c. Let ice melt; *do not* use sharp objects to remove ice.
   d. Remove melted ice.
   e. Replace foodstuffs.
   f. Turn freezer *on*.

Dishwashing Machine

1. Clean machine after each washing period. Remove bits of food and sediment caught in the openings.
2. *Weekly*: drain water from the machine and flush the inside; remove strainer trays and clean with a stiff brush. Do not allow scraps from the trays to get into the pump.

Ovens

1. Clean weekly.
2. Do not clean oven until it is cool.
3. If racks and shelves are removable, take out and clean. Remove encrusted material from them and from inside of oven with a blunt scraper or wire brush.
4. Clean heat control, but do not loosen or remove dials.
5. Clean outside of oven.

Dry Food Storage

1. Clean monthly.
2. Remove all foods from storage area.
3. Brush out all loose soil.
4. Wipe area with disinfectant solution.
5. Rinse with clean water.
6. Dry with clean cloth.

Drinking Fountains

Clean daily with disinfectant solution.

Washing Walls in the Kitchen

Walls need washing for the sake of appearance and for reasons of health. Dirty walls make rooms dark and dingy. If walls and ceilings are clean, germs cannot breed there, and risks for spreading disease are less. Dust and dirt collect on walls over long periods of time and form a greasy film, especially in places like kitchens where there is moisture and smoke. The way the walls should be cleaned depends on how dirty they are and what they are made of. Tile walls are nonabsorbent. They may be washed with a neutral cleaning solution and rinsed with a clean sponge and clear water. They are polished with a soft dry cloth. Graystone and cement walls are dusted with a stiff brush or washed according to directions. Use a neutral cleaning solution and rinse with clear water. Badly soiled walls should be soaked with muriatic solution, then rinsed with clear water. Let the walls dry overnight.

D2 — Dishwashing Procedures

Dish Sanitizing

Dishwashing may be done either manually or mechanically. Regardless of the equipment used, there are certain procedures that should be followed to ensure the proper washing and sanitizing of tableware and eating utensils. These procedures should be posted in the dishwashing area.

Manual Dishwashing

Employees assigned manual dishwashing duties should:

1. Be provided with appropriate and suitable equipment in which to wash the dishes and tableware. A three-compartment sink is required, or three dishpans.
2. Prescrape or preflush dishes and tableware before washing them to remove large particles of food and soil.
3. Use a sufficient amount of an effective detergent in hot water for dishwashing (wash in sink 1).
4. Rinse dishes and tableware thoroughly to remove detergent (rinse in sink 2).
5. Immerse dishes and tableware for at least 1/2 minute in clean hot water at a temperature of at least 170 degrees Fahrenheit to sanitize (sanitize in sink 3). OR
6. Immerse dishes in a sanitizing solution in the concentration, at the temperature, and for the length of time as recommended by the local health authority.
7. Allow dishes to air dry.

Mechanical Dishwashing

Employees assigned mechanical dishwashing duties should:

1. Be provided with mechanical dishwashing equipment of suitable size and capacity to wash dishes and other tableware within a reasonable length of time.
2. Be provided with mechanical dishwashing equipment that has thermometers that are in good workable condition and that can be easily read.
3. Be provided with the manufacturer's directions for operation and care of the dishwashing machine.
4. Prescrub or preflush dishes and tableware before washing them to remove large particles of food and soil.
5. Use a sufficient amount of dishwashing powder in the machine or dispenser to thoroughly clean dishes.
6. Keep wash water reasonably clean during the dishwashing period.

7. Have a wash water temperature of at least 140 degrees Fahrenheit, and in single tank conveyor machines, the wash water should be at least 160 degrees Fahrenheit.
8. Have a sanitizing final rinse water temperature of at least 180 degrees Fahrenheit at the entrance to the machine's manifold.

After dishwashing and sanitizing dishes and tableware, handle in such a manner as to protect them from contamination. Clean spoons, knives, and forks should be picked up by their handles. Clean bowls, cups, and glasses should be picked up so that fingers do not touch inside or lip surfaces. Clean and sanitized dishes and tableware should be stored above the floor in a clean, dry location and protected from splash, dust, and other contamination.

E. *Bookkeeping Procedures*

E1 — Receipts

Funds may be received from the following sources:

1. Client fees	All Centers
2. Client donations	All Centers
3. Contributions	All Centers

The following will be received only at the centers listed next to the source:

4. Craft Income	El Rinconcito, Sirrine
5. Meal Income	El Rinconcito
6. Revenue Sharing	El Rinconcito, Sirrine, Vista Nueva
7. Title III	Longview, Vista Nueva
8. Title XX	El Rinconcito, Sirrine, Vista Nueva
9. United Way	Sirrine
10. Scholarship Income	Sirrine, Prescott
11. In Kind Income	Longview, Vista Nueva

When funds are received, determine what the source is (see 1-11 above).

For all funds except *Client Donations*, follow this procedure:

1. Issue receipt in triplicate, give one copy each to:
   a. Person or agency making payment (Blue).
   b. FSL (Yellow).
   c. ADC Program (White).

NOTE: If a check is received, stamp "For Deposit Only" on the back *immediately*.

2. On all receipts write:
   a. Date.
   b. *Who* money was "Received From."
   c. What for (e.g., employee meals, client fees, etc.).
   d. Amount of payment.
   e. Specific designation:
      1) Client fees (fee payers).
      2) Contributions (e.g., crafts, employee meals).
   f. Account information if applicable:
      1) Amount of account.
      2) Amount paid.
      3) Balance.
   g. Information on "How Paid" (cash, check, M.O.).
   h. Signature of staff person receiving funds.

NOTE: Keep *all* checks and cash in the safe or locked file cabinet.

E2 — Donations

Client Donations

Client donations are those funds which are contributed by non-fee-paying clients.

The procedure is as follows:

1. When funds are donated, a client donation receipt is issued if the client requests one.
2. If the donation is by check, the check is stamped "for deposit only" on the back.
3. A record of the donations is kept in the *Client Donations Record* under the client's name.
   a. Date.
   b. Who made the donation (e.g., Public Fiduciary).
   c. Amount of the donation.
   d. Total amount donated to date.
   e. Receipt number (corresponds to #4 below).
4. Weekly, combine all client donation monies and make one receipt. Example: #0958 (see following examples).
5. Enter this amount in the weekly *Donation Ledger*.

Participant Donations — Collection of ADC Contributions

1. Each morning, an envelope will be attached to each participant's name badge. As the person arrives at the center, they will pick up their envelope along with their name badge. Their name will be on their envelope.
2. After the participants have placed their donations in their envelopes, the envelopes will be placed in a box marked Contributions at the secretary's desk.
3. Each day, the secretary will open each envelope and record each donation in a ledger. Each participant will have his own page in the ledger to record his donation.
4. Receipts will be given out at the end of the month for those that request one.
5. Daily totals will be kept on file.
6. Deposits will be made weekly or biweekly.

NOTE: Use discretion in collection of donations. For example: If the client's family donates once a month, don't give that participant a daily envelope. Use *good judgement*.

E3 — Deposits

1. Deposits should be made, at a minimum, weekly, and on the last day of the month.
2. All checks must be stamped "For Deposit Only."
3. The procedure for making a deposit is as follows:
   a. Use a preprinted FSL deposit slip, write in the ADC program name.
   b. Write the date.
   c. Count the currency and enter the total next to *Currency*.
   d. Count the coins and enter next to *Coins*.
   e. List each check separately — record the bank number (usually found in upper right hand corner of the check).
   f. Total the amounts and write the total at the bottom of the deposit slip.
   g. Make the deposit slip in triplicate:
      1) The original deposit slip and the money go to the bank.
      2) FSL gets one copy.*
      3) The ADC program keeps one copy.*

   *Both of these copies must have deposit detail written on them. See example:

Client Fees	$72.00
Client Donations	260.00
Crafts Sale	9.00

E4 — Client Fees

1. Hours of ADC participation are recorded daily on the *Client Billing Statement*. (Taken from the daily sign-in sheet or spread sheet.)
2. At the end of the month, the total amount due is tabulated, and a new balance is computed.
3. The billing statement is prepared in triplicate:
   a. White copy to FSL.
   b. Yellow copy remains at the ADC program.

    c. A xerox copy is sent to the client or their family.
4. When the account is paid, a receipt is issued showing:*
    a. Date.
    b. Client name and address.
    c. Amount paid.
    d. How paid.   ˙
    e. Staff person receiving the payment.
    f. Length of billing period.

*Be sure to put on the receipt: *Client Fees*.

5. Mail the receipt to person responsible for the client's account.*

**Use good judgement* — Many family members pay the fee and *do not* want the bill given to the participant!

E5 — Posting on Spread Sheet

1. Each day the secretary of the ADC checks the following sheets:
    a. Participant sign-in/sign-out (ADC-15).
    b. Nutritional Supplementation (ADC-17).
    c. Transportation:
      1) DES Sheet (if applicable), and
      2) Daily transportation form (ADC-16).
2. Once it is determined that the sheets are correct and complete, the following totals are tabulated and noted at the top of the sheets:
    a. Participant units of service.
    b. Meals served.
    c. Van trips.
3. The sheets are then given to the director who proofreads the sheets and checks the totals and then initials it.
4. The secretary then posts the totals on the spread sheets (ADC-02 and ADC-04).

E6 — Petty Cash

1. Do not keep more than $100.00 in petty cash at any time. Purchases totaling more than $100.00 must be ap-

proved by the corporate ADC Field Director and typed on a Purchase Requisition.
2. The petty cash fund should be kept in a locked file cabinet, safe, etc.
3. A limited number of people should have access to the fund for accountability purposes.
4. Remember to record *all* purchases, reimbursements, and requests for reimbursements on *Petty Cash Claim* (DF3-80). Use a carbon, make two copies (keep one at the center).

Purchases

1. Write the date.
2. Under *Description*, record the name of the item purchased/where it was purchased. Example: punch balls/ K-Mart.
3. Record the amount of the purchase in the correct column. Example: Activities/Rec.
4. Calculate the balance remaining and enter in the *Balance* column.
5. Attach receipts to *Petty Cash Claim*. ADC Program Director must sign and date all receipts. ALL purchases must have receipts turned in.

Deposits

1. Write the date.
2. Under *Description*, write "Reimbursement" and the amount.
3. Under *Balance*, record the new balance.

Request for Reimbursement

1. Write the date.
2. Under *Description*, write "Request for Reimbursement" and the amount requested.
3. Do not let your petty cash get too low. Send in Request when you have spent $25.00.

4. Be sure that the amount of request balances out with the amount of petty cash your center is approved for (e.g., $100.00).
5. The ADC Corporate Field Director and the ADC Program Director must approve all *Petty Cash Claims*.
6. Send one copy to FSL and keep one copy at the ADC.

Cash Advances

If a cash advance is taken from the petty cash fund, a *Received of Petty Cash* slip must be filled out.

1. Write the date.
2. Next to "For" write what will be purchased.
3. Next to "Charge to" write name of account to be charged (e.g., Ed. & Rec. Supplies).
4. The person receiving the money must sign for it.
5. When the purchase is made and a receipt presented, this *Received of Petty Cash* form is discarded.

PETTY CASH CLAIM

DATE	WHERE BOUGHT-DESCRIPTION	POSTAGE	PRINTING	OFFICE SUPPLIES	EDUCA. RECREA. SUPPLIES	CUSTOD. MAINT. SUPPLIES	OTHER SUPPLIES IDENTIFY	FOOD	TRAVEL CONF. & MEETINGS	MISC.	BALANCE
		$	$	$	$	$	$	$	$	$	$

E7 - Petty Cash Claim

F. Social Services

F1 — Summary of Procedures for ADC Participants

1. Social worker makes contact with participant and family, interviews and does a work-up on all forms.
2. Doctor's form is sent to the named doctor and received back at the ADC office. If not received within two weeks, a follow-up phone call should be made. Family should be encouraged to follow through to obtain medical forms.
3. Entire work-up reviewed by ADC staff by holding a case conference.
4. The family and possible participant is notified of the decision.
5. Documentation must be filed as to why/why not a possible participant is either accepted or rejected.
6. Social worker will advise all staff as to the new participant's arrival.
7. Notify transportation coordinator to make transportation arrangement if using center's transportation.
8. *Follow Procedures for New Participant* (see special procedures in sections B.3. and C.5.).
9. Complete monthly progress notes.
10. Participant will be staffed at 3-, 4-, or 6-month intervals.
11. Social worker completes *Six Month Narrative Summary*.
12. Upon closure, social worker completes *Closing Narrative*.

F2 — Assessment Procedure*

1. The purpose of the initial assessment is to determine if the client is suitable for adult day care.
2. At the time of initial assessment, discuss ADC with family and client.
3. Prior to or during the assessment, obtain income information. If client is Title XX or Title III eligible and

ADC is Title XX or Title III funded, refer the person to Maricopa County Department of Health Services case management. The participant or family must call. The phone number is 267-5282.

*Keep a record to insure the referral does not get lost in the process.Call family back if referral does not come through.

4. Use the following forms to assess functional level of the client:
   a. White — County Medical assessment form.
   b. Orange — Day care assessment packet:
      1) Social history,
      2) Care assessment,
      3) Life satisfaction index, and
      4) Scoring sheet (may be synonymous with intake, depending on the participant).
5. Reassure client that "this is not a test."
6. After assessment, tell client that we will "be in touch with them." *Make no promises regarding acceptance in ADC.*

F3 - Social History Assessment

SOCIAL HISTORY

NAME:_____ WORKER:_____

D.O.B.:_____ DATE:_____

REASON FOR REFERRAL:_____

_____

_____

PHYSICAL DESCRIPTION:_____

_____

_____

BACKGROUND:_____

_____

_____

PRESENT SITUATION: _____

_____

_____

IMPRESSIONS AND RECOMMENDATIONS: _____

_____

_____

_____

_____

_____

_____

_____

_____

F4 - Physical Assessment

Client Name _____

VII. PHYSICAL ASSESSMENT

Check if   **F I N D I N G S**

W H L		
___	General Appearance	
	Height, Weight, Hygiene	
___	BP P R T	
	Pulmonary	
___	SOB, COPD, IB, Pneumonia	
	Cough, Dyspnea	
	Cardiovascular	
___	43P, irregular beats, murmur, Angina,	
	history of M.I., varicosities,	
	peripheral vascular disease	
	Integumentary	
___	Skin color & temp., vascularity,	
	turgor, lesions, edema	
	Endocrine	
___	Diabetes, thyroid	
	Neurological	
___	Reflexes, gait, tremors, history	
	of CVA, epilepsy, DT's, trauma	
	Musculoskeletal	
___	Arthritis, amputations, muscular	
	atrophy, chronic pain, spinal	
	deformity, history of injury	
	Gastrointestinal	
___	Appetite, ulcers, hepatitis, CB,	
	weight loss, blood in stools, diarrhea,	
	constipation, incontinence	

<u>Genitourinary</u>
Stones, infection, VD, incontinence

___

<u>EENT</u>
Vision acuity, hearing acuity,
mucous membrane, gums, dental

___

VIII. SUMMARY OF SITUATION AND NEEDS

DEGREE OF FUNCTIONAL IMPAIRMENT:
___None
___Mild Problem
___Moderate Problem
___Severe Problem
___Totally Impaired

Worker's rating of Client's overall
need for service:
___No Need   ___Mild Need
___Moderate Need ___Severe Need
___Desperate Need

Case Mgr:_____
Date:_____
Comm Hlth Nrs:_____
Date:_____

FOR USE BY MARICOPA COUNTY DEPT. OF HEALTH SERVICES AND CITY OF PHOENIX HUMAN RESOURCE DEPT.

F5 — Client Intake

NOTE: Intake may be started at the time of assessment (if client is completely appropriate). Once the person has been staffed and determined to be appropriate for ADC:

1. Determine the hourly/daily rate for ADC.
2. Schedule times for participation.
   a. Should be a minimum of two days a week, four hours a day.
   b. Stress that the schedule must be adhered to unless the change is discussed beforehand with the ADC staff.
3. Discuss transportation arrangements.
   a. Families are to provide transportation for the participant.
   b. If the participant has no family or they are unable to provide transportation, contact other sources such as Red Cross.
4. Use the following forms:
   a. Intake Fact Sheet.
   b. Day Care Payment Contract.

    c. Participation Agreement (optional). (Use when there is a problem. *This form can be threatening* to the client and family.)

    d. Medical Release (signed by the participant and to be sent to the personal physician).

    e. Health Review.

5. Obtain a social history of the client.
    a. Name.
    b. Birthdate.
    c. Reason for referral.
    d. Physical description.
    e. Background.
    f. Impressions.
    g. Recommendations.

F6—Staffing Procedure

Initial staffing (must be *prior* to participant acceptance).

1. Use the *Case Staffing Report*.
2. Relate Social History.
3. Prepare a Care Plan:
    a. Form objectives.
    Example: 1) Assess as to abilities (initial staffing),
    2) Restore bladder control, and
    3) Monitor health.
    b. List strategies.
    c. Select one staff person to be responsible for each objective.

Staffing Schedule

1. Initial staffing will occur before acceptance.
2. Follow-up staffing—two-week intervals following initial staffing:
    a. Review progress towards objectives.
    b. Discuss new problems.
    c. Determine date for next staffing (3, 4, 6 months).
3. Subsequent staffings:
    a. Discuss progress towards objectives.

b. Discuss new problems.

c. Make any necessary revisions.

F7 — Progress Notes

1. Must be completed monthly on each participant.
2. May be completed by director or assigned ADC staff, and kept in participant's file.
3. Be sure to date entry and staff must sign full name and position he/she occupies, e.g., 3/15/83 Joe Smith/Social Worker

F8 — Narratives

Six-Month Narrative

1. Must be completed every six months by social worker.
2. Remains in participant's file.

Closing Narrative

1. Must be completed at case closure by social worker.
2. Place in participant's file and file under "Inactive Participants."

Adult Day Care Contact Sheet

1. Completed by social worker.
2. Kept in participant's file.

G. *Health Surveillance*

1. Each adult day care participant should have a current *Medical Report* on file. This report must be filled out by the participant's physician and should contain information regarding:
   a. History of any illnesses.
   b. Susceptibility.
   c. Special requirements for health and maintenance.
   This (a, b, and c) must be documented in the participant's file.

2. Each treatment administered to an ADC participant *must* be recorded and documented in the participant's file.
3. Participant's physical health should be continually observed for any changes. Records of blood pressure and pulse rate must be documented on the *Vital Signs Form*. Entry in the participant's file should be made as often as required, but at a minimum, once a month.
4. Coordinate with the community agencies to assure that the participant is receiving the proper medical care on the day or time that the participant is not at ADC. Be sure to document which community agencies are providing services.
5. Assist the participant with administration of medication only with instructions from issuing physician or pharmacist. Instructions for medications must be kept in participant's file.

G1 — Health Monitoring

1. Be alert to subtle changes as well as gross changes in a participant's physical conditions:
   a. Increased sleepiness.
   b. Increased anxiety/agitation.
   c. Change in personality.
   d. Change in level of personal hygiene.
   e. Loss of appetite
   f. Increased difficulty in ambulation
   g. Incontinence.

These changes may indicate the presence of health problems which require a physician's attention. Notify the family of the participant and/or contact the participant's physician.

H. *Adult Day Care Activities*

Each adult day care center's activity program is as different as its participants and as innovative as its staff's creativity. Though certain activities are basic to every program, the variety of activities is largely determined by the participants' needs, abilities, and interests. Every program day is, however, structured and purposeful. The purpose of the day care center's program is to provide therapeutic and rehabilitative activities for its participants. An awareness of the frailty of the elderly and their functional activities is important in deciding what activities are to be offered at what times during the day.

The major considerations in activity planning are:

1. Participant/staff involvement.
2. Equal spacing of meals and snacks.
3. Maximum energy activities in the morning.
4. Alternating activity with quiet times.

Activities

1. A *Daily Schedule* should be prepared by the activity coordinator and posted where participants will see it.
2. A *Monthly Schedule* should be prepared by the 25th of the preceding month. This schedule is posted on the first day of the month. Include *Special Events*, *holidays*, and *birthdays*.
3. Resources for activities can be found at:
   a. The public library (films, slides, records).
   b. The entertainment file kept at each center.
   c. Other adult day care centers.
4. Aim to provide age appropriate activities. Remember, the participants are *adults*, not children. Most activities can be adapted to varying functional levels. Some good activities are:
   a. Table games, card games, word games.
   b. Films, slide presentations.
   c. Small and large group discussions.
   d. Current events.
   e. Cooking, food experiences.
   f. Health and hygiene presentations.
   g. Usable craft projects (weaving, handwork, sewing, wood working).
   h. Sing-alongs.
   i. Exercise (using appropriate motions and safeguards).

    j. Reality orientation (sensory retraining for special participants).

    k. Range of motion (stroke victims).

5. Participation in all activities is *highly encouraged*, but never use bodily force. Participants are required to join the group for lunch and exercise.

H1 — Guidelines for Screening Adult Day Care Entertainment

Entertainment provided for adult day care participants should be appropriate to the backgrounds and interests of the older people. It also should respond to sensory losses, changed intellectual abilities, and comfort needs. The following rules can be helpful:

1. The content of the entertainment should be familiar or relate to familiar experiences of the audience. For example, old familiar songs, well-known classical music, and traditional plays may be very effective.
2. Plots should be simple, involve few players, and be easy to follow. People who have visual, auditory, or mental impairments can find it difficult to keep track of many characters and complex plots.
3. The style of presentation should be familiar. Some clever and modern productions, such as those involving actors who change hats and voices and play more than one character or actors remaining visible onstage when the character they play is supposed to be elsewhere, may not make sense to elderly people.
4. Speakers or actors should have clear, easy to understand voices; high or soft voices are poor.
5. The pace of the performance should not be too fast. Older people need a bit more time to process and understand verbal and visual messages.
6. The visual portion of the performance should convey enough meaning and provide enough entertainment to hold the interest of severely hard-of-hearing people. Acting that has almost a pantomime quality about it and dancing or movement to accompany music are particularly effective.

7. Performers should be encouraged to wear clothing or costumes that will contrast with the background where they will be performing. For example, if the background is dark wood paneling, a singer must be easy to see in white or yellow. One particularly enjoyable "show" was put on by two singers who wore pretty, long dresses, one red and one white. The audience enjoyed their attractive appearance, and they were able to see them well against a dark background.

8. The "stage" should be relatively uncluttered with people. A few characters at a time are easiest to see and follow.

9. Sound effects should be avoided if possible. Background music and sound effects may interfere with hearing voices.

10. The basic plot, format, outline, or program should be provided in advance so nursing home staff can prepare residents for what to expect and to appreciate and understand the performance.

11. Entertainers who have had much adult day care or nursing home experience may have the ability to elicit audience participation by calling for clapping or hand raising. For example, "This next song is for everyone who grew up on a farm. How many of you grew up on a farm?" When the entertainers are not experienced, the staff members can make announcements and introductions to establish an atmosphere for enjoying the entertainment.

12. It is important for entertainers to have some knowledge and respect for aging adult day care participants. Even if they are well-meaning, condescending attitudes and underestimation of the intellectual abilities and mental status of residents can be damaging. These things might be clarified in the initial phone contact, or a 20- to 30-minute meeting to arrange the entertainment might be used as a time to help entertainers learn appropriate attitudes and approaches.

13. Entertainers who are known to the participants can be

especially effective. Employees who have talents can provide great enjoyment to residents who enjoy seeing a new side of a familiar face.

14. Entertainment should not be too long because many residents will not be comfortable sitting for long periods of time.

(Source: *Ebenezer Center for Aging Minneapolis, MN*)

H2 — Typical Exercises Used in a Group Setting

Breathing

1. Raise arms forward and up, breathing in. Lower arms sidewards and down, breathing out.
2. Hands clasped on top of head, breathe in raising chest, breathe out while relaxing.
3. Arms straight and held at sides, breathe in rolling arms out, breathe out as arms relax.
4. Hands behind the neck, breathe in as elbows move back.

Pectoral Stretch

1. Row your boat.
2. Hands behind neck, move elbows back.
3. Breast stroke.

Face and Neck Exercises

1. Head circling.
2. Chew gum.
3. Pull head high with chin in.
4. Blow bubbles — actual bubbles may be blown from commercial supplies at party stores or grocery stores. This exercise may be combined with deep breathing exercises.

Arm Exercises

1. Clench fist.
2. Throw baseball.
3. Throw basketball from chest.
4. Bounce ball from overhead.
5. Arms forward and upward with elbows straight, lower sidewards and down.
6. Bat the ball.
7. Hands to shoulder, overhead, to shoulder, then down.
8. "Yes, we have no bananas."
9. Arms at sides, elbows straight, roll arms out.
10. Turn palms up and down.
11. Swimming—the breast stroke, back stroke, slow "butterfly."

Leg and Ankle Exercises (sitting)

1. Ankle circling.
2. Ice curling.
3. Alternate knee straightening.
4. Alternate knee to chest.
5. Marching.

Leg and Ankle Exercises (sitting or standing)

1. Mark time—tapping on the floor.
2. Rock up on toes, then on heels.
3. Alternate knees to chest, if possible. Use hands to assist.
4. Kick with knee straight.
5. Marching—grand right and left to a rhythm band.

Back Exercises (sitting or standing)

1. Row.
2. Hands on hips, twist first one way then the other.
3. Hands at sides, reach for knees.
4. "Tick Tock"
5. "Wheelchair push-ups": hands on arms of chair, feet

on floor, lift buttocks off the chair momentarily (lock the wheelchair!). This is where added staff can be of great help so that patients can each try this.

Results Anticipated

1. Strengthening of weakened muscle groups.
2. Gradual loosening of contractures.
3. Increased vital capacity.
4. Improved posture.
5. Increased socialization of patients.
6. Less cathartics and less narcotics.
7. Improved gait.
8. Closer relationship between patients and staff.
9. Less daydreaming and hallucinating.
10. Better grooming, especially when this is commented upon by the leader in a positive way.
11. Group spirit which can be carried over into other activities.

It cannot be overemphasized that having a good time is essential. Special refreshments once a week are fun, as are any and all ideas for providing the residents with fun and motivation for the positive side of life.

I. *Volunteers*

I1 — Guidelines for Volunteers in a Recreation Program for the Elderly

The use of volunteers in recreation programs requires attention to all the previously delineated aspects of a volunteer program. Assignments given to volunteers in recreation programs may be chosen from any of the following areas:

a. *Administrative or advisory help,* usually involving responsibilities on boards, councils, or committees or tasks, such as carrying out surveys of recreation interests;

b. *Group leadership*, involving a direct role in designing, organizing and carrying out various program activities;
c. *Non-leadership roles*, such as officiating at events, and furnishing transportation;
d. *Clerical or maintenance work* including registering participants and other office duties; and
e. *Miscellaneous services*, such as preparing publicity material, participating as a guest speaker or providing other needed expertise.

(Kraus, 1981)

Specific activities in which volunteers in a recreation program for the elderly could assist in are:

1. Leading special groups such as current events, travel, reminiscing, writing, and gardening.
2. Assisting the recreation leaders in the arts and crafts program.
3. Assisting in reality therapy groups.
4. Accompanying residents on special outings and to events such as dances, dinners, and parties.

Another important role of volunteers in adult day care recreation programs is that of providing entertainment for the residents. It is important that the entertainment be appropriate and of good quality. The entertainment needs to be screened and any necessary adaptations made to insure that presentations are appropriate.

Staff-Volunteer Relations

As noted before, a good rapport is necessary between volunteers and paid staff. Volunteer staff are not a replacement for paid staff. The volunteer needs to understand the differences in responsibility between staff and volunteer positions. If a particular staff person is unwilling to supervise volunteers, volunteers should not be assigned to that individual.

Assessment of Performance

Volunteers *need to know if they are doing a good job*. This feedback can be in the form of verbal reports or more formal semiannual written evaluations. The more frequent the evaluation, regardless of how informal it is, the more likely the duties and responsibilities of the volunteer will be kept current. The following points are suggested to help keep volunteer motivation high:

1. Volunteers must not be taken for granted.
2. Time should be taken to discover a volunteer's strengths and weaknesses.
3. Volunteers must see the relationship of their job to the total effort and importance of their contribution.
4. Volunteers *work best in a friendly atmosphere* where their *efforts are obviously needed and appreciated*.
5. Volunteer's work should be regularly assessed to make sure they are neither overworked nor underworked.
6. Volunteers should receive as much encouragement and feedback as possible.
7. Volunteers need to be informed on the organization as a whole.
8. Volunteers need to be consulted and asked for ideas and suggestions.

Due to the short duration of many volunteer assignments, formal written evaluations may be unsuitable. In that case, informal evaluation assumes a greater role.

When Volunteers Arrive:

1. Greet them!
2. Have them sign-in.
3. Give them a name badge.
4. Give them a meaningful task.

When Volunteers Leave:

1. Thank them!!
2. Have them sign-out.

3. Keep the name badges at the ADC Center.
4. Thank them again!!

I2 — Foundation for Senior Living

Adult Day Care Center Policies for Volunteers

1. The purpose of the center is to offer the opportunity for the elderly and physically disabled participants to maintain or increase independent functioning in an atmosphere where friendships can develop. Volunteers will help work toward these goals by treating each participant with respect and dignity. Volunteers should not wait on participants, but should encourage them to help themselves and each other.
2. Each participant will be recognized as an individual having different feelings, opinions, knowledge, talents, and skills gained through varied life experiences and cultural heritages. Each participant will be accepted for what he/she is and for what their culture expects them to be.
3. A volunteer's attitude should be one of sharing with and learning from the participants. Volunteers should not offer any medical counsel.
4. All personal information learned about the individual participants will be kept strictly confidential; i.e., between each volunteer involved and the staff at the center.
5. In order that the time a volunteer spends at the center be most useful, each volunteer will come in on a regular basis, at a time agreed upon by the volunteer and the center's director. The block of time spent at the center will be spent as the director and volunteer agree. Volunteers will be faithful in carrying out these duties.
6. If a volunteer cannot come in at the agreed upon time, the volunteer will notify the center as soon as she/he knows that she/he cannot come to the center.
7. Volunteers should keep open minds and be willing to do things the way they are instructed. They will work in

harmony with the staff and be willing to share their knowledge and experience with the staff.

8. Volunteers have a right to know about the center, its policies, its organization, and its program.
9. Each volunteer has the right to be treated as a co-worker and have an appropriate job assignment with consideration for preference, experience, education, and availability.
10. Each volunteer has the right to scheduled conferences with his or her staff supervisor. Suggestions will be heard, appreciated, and considered.
11. Each volunteer has the right to training, guidance, and instruction in working with the elderly.
12. As a volunteer at the center, she/he will also benefit from the deep feeling of satisfaction which comes through sharing with others, and helping others to help themselves.

I have read and understand the above policies.

Volunteer_____

13 - Volunteer Registration Form

VOLUNTEER REGISTRATION

DATE _____

TELEPHONE _____

NAME _____

ADDRESS_____
city　　　　state　　zip

I heard about _____ Center at, on, or from

_____

OCCUPATION _____

PREV. OCCUPATIONS _____

CURRENT OR PREV. VOLUNTEER WORK _____

AREAS OF EDUCATION _____

HOBBIES_____ LANGUAGES_____

I am a full year resident _____   Part-time resident _____

Times I will be available _____
                                            (days, hours, etc.)

Period will serve _____

Are there any physical limitations? _____

In emergency, contact: NAME:_____

                        ADDRESS:_____

                        PHONE: _____

        I want to be a volunteer at _____ Center because

        _____

        _____

        _____

MISC. INFORMATION.

I4 - Volunteer Agreement Form

VOLUNTEER AGREEMENT

I want to be a Volunteer in Adult Day Care because:

_____

_____

_____

_____

I am willing to do a variety of things as the Staff directs me in accordance with my capabilities.

I accept the responsibility of being on time on the days assigned to me.

In case of an emergency and I cannot come in, I will call the day ahead.

I will regard personal matters at the Center as confidential.

I know the Center is new, the Staff is new, and consequently everything is not perfect. I will strive to learn and grow with them.

I realize that the role of a Volunteer is an extremely important one. Without Volunteers, the Center could not function. I will be proud to be accepted. My duties may involve some of the following:

> Morning Greetings - helping with exercises - serving snacks - group discussions - one-to-one conversations - reading - going for a walk - pushing wheelchairs - holding a hand - helping in the bathroom - arts and crafts - cleanup - maintenance - clerical work - telephoning - card playing - bingo - checkers - dominos - dancing - explaining

entertainment to a blind person – helping with new programs as they are put into action.

Name _____

Address _____

Telephone _____

Hours and days available _____

J. *Personal Hygiene*

J1 – Bathroom Accidents

1. Handle the situation with tact. Do not call undue attention to the problem.
2. The staff person discovering the situation is responsible for handling it. Do not delegate.
3. Try to reach the participant's family. Explain the situation and ask them to come to the center and clean up the participant or take him/her home.
4. If the family cannot be reached, follow this procedure:
   a. Assist the person in removing soiled clothing and cleaning themselves. Keep your attitude light and helpful, not condescending.
   b. Substitute clean clothing for the soiled clothing. Place the soiled clothing in a plastic bag with the participant's name on it (to be sent home).
   c. Clean the bathroom area, if necessary. Use a disinfectant solution to wipe the toilet and floor area.

J2 – Personal Appearance

If a participant arrives at the center in an inappropriate condition (bad odor, soiled clothing, soiled hair and/or body):

1. Take the participant into a room away from the group – *be discreet.*
2. Call the family or group home and notify them of the situation. Ask them to come to the center and take the participant home.

3. If the family or group home cannot be reached, try to correct the situation. Continue trying to contact the family.
4. If the situation persists, consult with the social worker.

K. *Monthly Reports*

K1 — Monthly Reports Due to FSL

A copy of each report is on file at the Foundation for Senior Living.

1. Spread Sheets for Title III, Title XX and Feepayers (ADC- 03).
2. ADC Monthly Report (Buff) (ADC-04)
3. Billing (Individual Client)
4. Activity Report (ADC-06)
5. Monthly Summary Sheet 16 (b) (2) Vehicle (Green) (ADC-07)
6. Vehicle Checklist (ADC-08)
7. Monthly Repairs on Vehicle (ADC-09)
8. Staff/Volunteer Meal Report (ACC-10) (pink) keep at center.
9. Catered Meal Report (ADC-11)
10. Kitchen Cleaning Report (ADC-12)
11. Donation Collections Report (ADC-14)
12. Space Status Report (ADC-19)
13. A.A.A. Region 1 Monthly Social Service Report (ADC-37)

K2 — Copies of Reports to ADC Corporate Field Director

1. ADC Monthly Report (ADC-04)
2. Activity Report (ADC-06)
3. Catered Meal Report (ADC-11)
4. Kitchen Cleaning Report (ADC-12)
5. Donation Report and Chart (ADC-14)
6. A.A.A. Region 1 Monthly Social Service Report (ADC-37)

7. Advisory Board's Minutes and Agenda
8. Meetings Attended by Director
9. Fire Drill Report (four times a year)
10. Monthly Report for FSL President/CEO
11. Space Status Report (ADC-19)

ALL *invoices* and *deposits* must be *sent in promptly*.

K3 — Reports to Stay at Centers

1. Participant sign-in/sign-out sheet (ADC-15)
2. Daily Transportation Form (ADC-16)
3. Nutritional Supplementation Daily Participation Sign-In Sheet (ADC-17)
4. Interoffice Memo (ADC-18)
5. Space Status Report/FSL (ADC-19)
6. ADC Payment Contract (ADC-20)
7. Release of Medical Information (ADC-21)
8. Participation Agreement (ADC-22)
9. Intake Sheet (ADC-23)
10. Care Assessment (ADC-24)
11. Progress Notes (ADC-29)
12. Six Month Narrative Summary (ADC-30)
13. Closing Narrative (ADC-31)
14. Health Review (ADC-32)
15. Vital Signs (ADC-33)
16. Continence Retraining Schedule (ADC-35)
17. ADC Care Plan (ADC-36)

L.   Position Descriptions

L1 - Program Director

FOUNDATION FOR SENIOR LIVING

Position Title: Program Director
Department: FSL Program & Services

Position Summary:

Reports to Field Director of Adult Day Care; administers Adult Day Care program for the frail elderly; responsibility for intake and termination of clients; coordinates components which comprise five day week program; staff hiring, supervising, evaluating and terminating; prepares and monitors budget; markets fee paying programs, complies with policies and procedures of FSL; works with FSL programs and services Advisory Committee; cooperates with community agencies; maintains program facility and equipment; performs other job-related tasks deemed necessary and/or assigned by Field Director of Adult Day Care.

Key Duties and Responsibilities:

Administers daily program for frail elderly who require care and supervision by ensuring that required number of personnel is on duty by developing a written staffing schedule; assurance of client super-vision at all times; develops staff skills for working with the frail elderly; sends staff to training sessions, including CPR and transfer techniques; and team effort is encouraged by regular staff meetings; assures the quality care and supervision appropriate to client needs.

Responsible for final approval for client intake and termination. Pre and post admission conferences with staff as well as regular case conference to determine participants progress.

Coordinates recreation, socialization, health, transportation and social service components of Adult Day Care by ensuring that monthly calendar of events is posted and activities are appropriate to level of participant's functioning and interest; that weekly menus are posted and have been approved for nutritional value; meals are pre-pared and served to comply with government regulations; ensuring that client's physical and mental health are maintained by health person-nel; assuring safe transportation and/or suggesting alternatives for bringing clients to and from program by providing information; and referral to social services to client and the client's family.

Hires, supervises, evaluates, and terminates staff while complying with FSL Personnel policies and procedures; provides accurate job descriptions; maintains chronologicals; monitors employee hours and signs timesheets; authorizes mileage reimbursements, maintenance, and petty cash requests.

Prepares and monitors budgets, and works with FSL Administration in order to maintain zero deficit position ensuring that expenses do not exceed actual income level; maintains accurate accounts of expenses.

Effort:

May spend considerable portion of the day sitting at desk; also moves about throughout the facility; occasionally may need to assist with transfer of participant to and from wheelchair.

<u>Working Conditions:</u>

Works in a clean, well-lighted, well-heated and in the summer, air-conditioned office. Minimal noise from office machines and has own desk and telephone at which work is completed.

<u>Number of Employees Supervised:</u>

Directly - 8 or more.

Acceptance and understanding

_____
    employee signature

_____
         date

L2 - RN - Center Health Coordinator

FOUNDATION FOR SENIOR LIVING
Position Description

<u>Position Title:</u> RN - Center Health Coordinator
<u>Department:</u> Programs & Services ADC

<u>Position Summary:</u>

Reports to Program Director. Responsible for monitoring health of participants - liaison between health professionals; assumes leadership role in emergencies, does medical follow-up on participants; provides health education to staff, participants and their families; maintains medical supplies, interprets dietary needs; writes nursing recertification; participates in case conferences; maintains a record of treatments and medications; reports safety hazards; performs any other job-related duties deemed necessary and/or assigned by Program Director.

<u>Key Duties and Responsibilities:</u>

Monitors health condition of the participants in the day care program, which includes taking and documenting in case record, participants vital signs and noting and reporting any changes.

Serves as a liaison between health professionals and center staff. This is to include ensuring that there is a current medical report from participants own physician on each participant; maintaining an open flow of communication between the participant's physician and the center, ensuring accurate information is related to physician and that medical appointments are made and kept. Develops a written plan to be followed on each participant in the event of an emergency. Assumes the leadership role in all health emergency situations, calling paramedics when necessary and ensuring that everything possible is being done for the participant.

Educates the participants, families and staff in interpreting diagnosis and orders, assisting them to accept limitations and live with conditions when total rehabilitation is not possible. Maintains adequate amount of medical and nursing supplies.

Writes nursing recertification every 3 months. Participants monthly progress notes are taken from their case records and compiled for this report.

Actively participates as a team member in case conferences; this includes presenting medical information, giving input, writing down suggestions and following through on goals and objectives as established by the team.

Maintains a record of all treatments or medications administered at the center, making sure any medication administered at the center has written instruction of the participant's own personal physician.
Always performs in a professional manner as dictated by the code of ethics of the nursing profession and a representative of FSL.

L3 - Activity Coordinator

FOUNDATION FOR SENIOR LIVING
Position Description

Position Title: Activity Coordinator
Department: Program & Services ADC

Position Summary:

Reports to Program Director. Responsible for development of monthly calendar; design and implement the daily schedule; ensure that all planned activities are implemented; analyze the activity needs of the participants and develop programs to meet those needs; actively participate in case conference; observe and report significant changes in behavior; write progress notes; make purchases; carry through on care plans; maintain activity area; maintain an enthusiastic and positive attitude and flexibility; perform other job-related duties deemed necessary and/or assigned by Program Director.

Key Duties and Responsibilities:

Develop and submit within five days prior to the end of the calendar month an imaginative and varied monthly calendar of special events which will include birthday parties, holidays, participants' council (community meetings), field trips, speakers, entertainment, films. These scheduled events must be interesting to the participants and designed to meet their individual needs in the area of education, socialization, physical and mental development.

Design and implement daily schedules of activities; should include daily exercise program, reality orientation, individual and group crafts, discussion groups, activities of daily living; ensuring that the daily schedule is varied with respect to physical, mental and social activities to ethnic/racial interest and to level of participants functioning.

Actively participate in Case Conference; this includes giving input, writing down suggestions and following through on goals and objectives as established by the team.

Supervise all aides and volunteers ensuring that planned activities are implemented; gives directions to these workers and orients them to the activities program.

Observe behavior and note in participants' charts and reports to the Program Director or Health Coordinator the physical or attitude changes in the participants.

Write progress notes on monthly basis or as required by Program Director ensuring that they are written in a professional manner following the proper guidelines for progress notes. Maintain a confidential nature of all case records.

Responsible for making both minor and major activity purchases, ensuring that there are enough materials on hand so that programs can be carried out as planned minimizing the need for last minute purshases. May be required to be responsible for petty cash.

L4 - Groupworker/Program Aide

FOUNDATION FOR SENIOR LIVING
Position Description

Position Title: Groupworker/Program Aide
Department: Programs & Services ADC

Position Summary:

Reports to Activity Coordinator. Required to lead or assist in group discussion, reality orientation, daily exercise or craft group; may be required to write progress notes or attend Case Conference; keep day care area clean; maintain confidentiality; assist participants with meals and in washroom or with transferring; may be trained to take participants' blood pressure and weight; must be courteous to participants and staff and flexible in relation to all duties. Performs any other job-related tasks deemed necessary and/or assigned by Activity Coordinator.

Key Duties and Responsibilities:

May be required to either lead or assist in group discussion. Topics should be interesting to participants, and appropriate to their functioning level.

May be required to lead a reality orientation program or assist staff team in a 24-hour reality orientation; constantly reminding participants of place, time, date, and other recent important information.

As assigned, lead or assist in daily exercise class. Exercises should be fun, stimulating but not too strenuous; should promote increased flexibility; strength and endurance.

Assists participants with their arts and crafts; shows participants different techniques such as embroidery, crochet, flower-making, etc. These techniques are taught through demonstrations, participants then attempt techniques while worker monitors and corrects mistakes.

As assigned, program aide may be required to write program notes or attend case conferences; instructions will be provided in both of these areas by either Activity Coordinator or center's Social Worker.

Keeps all activity areas and washrooms neat and picked up because of spill and accidnets; may be required to do some heavier cleaning or mopping.

Maintains confidentiality with all participant's personal related matters at all times. Information may not be given out when requested by families, other participants, or unauthorized employees who do not have a need to know.

Helps with the serving of all food, assisting participants who need help and to help clean up as needed.

Assists participants in and out of van or private cars; also may be required to transfer participants to and from wheelchair to regular chair.

L5 - Social Worker

FOUNDATION FOR SENIOR LIVING
Position Description

Position Title: Social Worker
Department: Program & Services ADC

Position Summary

Reports to Program Director. Takes primary responsibility for determina-
tion of programmatic eligibility of potential Adult Day Care participants,
other than participants served by the Coordinated Services Systems; assists
in the development and carrying out of the Individual Program Plans (IPP)
for each person accepted into the Day Care Program; performs Casework
Services needed by the program participants; provides supportive services
to the families of the program participants; takes responsibility for case
records of each participant; participates with other center staff in
developing community awareness of adult day care programs and their benefits, including outreach work; performs any other job-related duties deemed
necesssary and/or assigned by Program Director.

Key Duties and Responsibilities

Takes primary responsibility for determinatidn of programmatic eligibility
of potential adult day care participants (other than participants served by
Coordinated Services System) by accepting all referrals; promptly conduct-
ing center's program and eligibility requirements for participation;
assessing participant's need for day care services, as well as programmatic
eligibility according to FSL guidelines and the participant's financial
responsibility; developing a social history on each applicant and presenting information regarding applicant at pre-admission case conference.

Assists in the development and carrying out of the Individual Program Plans
(IPP) by taking an active role in pre-admission case conference to determine acceptance of applicant; contributing to the development of social
service goals for each participant; administering the FSL care assessment
instrument within two weeks of admission and every six months thereafter
(other than participants served by the Coordinated Services System); taking
responsibility for the monitoring of the IPP's at case conferences on each
participant at least every six months.

Performs casework services needed by the program participants by assessing
participant's problems, strengths and weaknesses; setting social service
goals with the participant; providing counseling and/or support to participants to facilitate the prevention and allevaition of stress from psychosocial problems; intervening on behalf of the participant to foster access
to utilization of community resources and services for social support.
This is documented in Adult Day Care participant contact sheets.

Provides supportive services to the families of the program participants by
focusing on the total family system in order to support and strengthen
family unity; sharing with the family helpful suggestions and information
regarding care and support of the frail elderly; participation in planning
and implementation of family night sessions; providing support and/or
offering resources to families in crisis situations; provides training to
participants in family relations that are culturally, physically and age
appropriate, documenting this in adult day care contact sheets.

L6 - Secretary/Bookkeeper

FOUNDATION FOR SENIOR LIVING
Position Description

Position Title: Secretary/Bookkeeper
Department: Program & Services ADC

Position Summary:

Reports directly to Program Director. Performs all clerical duties related
to the center's operation; prepares daily and monthly reports; serves as an
information resource to people calling the center for information; provides
clerical assistance to other staff members as deemed necessary by the
Program Director; maintains daily attendance records; does billing for fee
payers; orders and maintains records of all purchases; answers the phone;
greets guests; types; makes photocopies; accounts for income; prepares
forms; maintains a well organized office; performs any other job-related
duties deemed necessary and/or assigned by Program Director.

Key Duties and Responsibilities:

Uses courtesy and proper manners over the telephone and in greeting anyone
who may come to the center seeking information; is responsive and helpful
as possible directing people to the appropriate staff; records messages
accurately ensuring the related messeages are directed to the appropriate
staff members as soon as possible.

Types all reports, papers, letters and memos as requested by the Program
Director and center staff; ensures that all typing is neat and accurate,
that all words are spelled correctly and sentences read smoothly.

Maintains daily attendance logs, including units of service, transportation
and meals; maintains all center files, including participant files, chrono-
logical correspondence file, tickler files, advisory board file, purchase
request book and all FSL day care forms ensuring that all files are continually updated and kept in an orderly fashion.

Interacts with the participants in a positive, friendly and helpful manner.
Maintains good working relationship with supervisor and nonsupervisory
staff.

Keeps an accurate account of all incoming money, including fees and payment
of staff meals. Makes weekly deposits of fee income. Keeps track of petty
cash ensuring an accurate balance between cash and receipts.

Prepares all necessary forms as requested; this will include but is not
limited to requests for printing, purchase requests, petty cash forms and
check request forms.

Is responsible for miscellaneous functions that constitute a well organized
office, such as ensuring that adequate brochures are available, that all
staff receive appropriate keys, that adequate office supplies are available
to staff, keeps office tidy.

Assists Activity Coordinator with scheduled events. Helps organize or
provides educational presentations of interest to seniors including but not
limited to entertainment, information, health and welfare items, and games,
parties, exercises, movies, etc. Will also assist participants in using
washroom.

Performance Requirements:

Job Knowledge:

Must have a chauffeurs license with an excellent driving record; be able to follow through on scheduled activities; able to head groups as well as to relate one-on-one. Know or be able to learn the proper transfer techniques as well as first-aid and CPR.

Experience:

Prior experience with frail elderly, driving experience and paid or volunteer experience working with crafts or leading group activities.

Effort:

Sits in van a good portion of the time. Will also be on feet leading groups and will be required to lift transferring participants.

Working Conditions:

Subject to heavy traffic and various weather conditions while driving to and from center; will work inside in a clean, well-lighted, well-heated in winter and air-conditions in summer building. Works with a high risk population. Must deal with potential life and death emergency situations, both at the center and in the van.

Number of Employees Supervised:

None.

Acceptance and understanding

_____
        employee signature

_____
             date

L7 - Transportation Coordinator/Groupworker

FOUNDATION FOR SENIOR LIVING
Position Description

Position Title: Transportation Coordinator/Groupworker
Department: Programs & Services ADC

Position Summary:

Reports to Program Director. Responsible for providing transportation for participants to and from center, keeping daily records and establishing a route, maintenance of van including cleaning and mechanical problems; follows all safety rules and emergency procedures and reports any problems; will assist Activity Coordinator with scheduled activities; performs any other job-related duties deemed necessary and/or assigned by Program Director.

Key Duties and Responsibilities:

Provides daily transportation for participants to and from the center in a safe and pleasant manner, using the center's van. Assists participants in and out of van.

Records daily transportation on appropriate forms, keeps track of time and mileage; also completes a monthly report.

Maintains accurate up-to-date client and daily report records. Makes sure all reports are completed accurately and on a timely basis. Each day completes a route for the following day, making sure route used is the best way to get the participants to and from the center.

Cleans interior and exterior by taking van to car wash once a month (more often if needed). In addition, keeps van filled with gas and is also aware of maintenance needs. Gets estimates and does leg work when mechanical problems arise getting approval from Director before repairs are made.

Follows all Arizona Department of Motor Vehicles' safety rules ensuring all seat belts are fastened prior to moving vehicle. Refrains from smoking, eating or drinking or participating in idle conversation while vehicle is in motion.

If emergency arises while transporting participants, follows the written emergency procedures, which include:

1. Do not leave the van unattended.
2. Raise hood and wait for someone to stop, ask them to call for help.
3. Administer any emergency first-aid.

Reports all participant absenteeism or incidents of any kind to center Social Worker or designated staff.

L8 - Maintenance Worker

FOUNDATION FOR SENIOR LIVING
Position Description

Position Title: Maintenance Worker
Department: Programs & Services ADC

Position Summary:

Reports to Program Director. Responsible for overall cleanliness, sanitation, and orderliness of the center facility; replenishes restroom, cleaning, and some sanitation supplies; helps with minor repair and upkeep. Performs any other job-related duties deemed necessary and/or assigned by Program Director.

Key Duties and Responsibilities:

Sweeps floors daily. Mops hallways, restrooms, and the dining area daily, and office rooms twice a week. Dry mops the dining room area with a sprayed mop to inhibit dust and then wet mops with antifungal agent.

Cleans restrooms, drinking fountains, ashtrays, wastebaskets, and lounge rooms daily. Places liners in wastebaskets when practical. Uses caution when emptying ashtrays to prevent fire hazard by emptying into a bucket containing water.   Cleans, as needed, miscellaneous equipment such as washing machine, air conditioning vents, and tools.   Prevents dirt build-up in any part of facility for health and safety reasons.

Vacuums facility daily.   Accomplishes dusting and general cleaning of furniture and woodwork on weekly basis.   Cleans windows and walls thoroughly at least once a month, or as needed.

Replenishes restrooms, cleaning, and some sanitation supplies as needed.

Helps with all minor repair and upkeep operations of the center.   For example: replacement of light bulbs and air conditioning filters.

Picks up outside litter, helping with the setting up of tables for meetings; keeping furniture in order; keeping equipment serviceable.

Performance Requirements:

Job Knowledge:

Worker should have experience in cleaning and maintaining building interiors.   Should have some knowledge of methods, materials, and equipment used in custodial work.   Must be able to work under moderate supervision and follow specific verbal and/or written directions for assigned tasks.   Needs perseverance in order to complete certain routine tasks that can be long and somewhat strenuous.   Must be able to work in cooperation with others in the completion of assigned tasks.

SCHEDULE 1, STAFFING WORKSHEET

FSAL Programs, Inc. for

AGENCY NAME

FOR PERIOD _____ TO _____

Page __1__ of __1__ pages

PREPARED BY/DATE

Pos. No.	Position Title and Employee Name	FTE	Total Salary For Contract Period	Total Salary Allocated to Services by Amount and % of Time										
				Day Care		$	%	$	%	$	%	$	%	$	%
1	Manager/Social Worker	1.0	$16,328. 100%	$16,328. 100%										
2	Registered Nurse	.63	8,000. 100%	8,000. 100%										
3	Aide	.50	4,500. 100%	4,500. 100%										
4	Activity Coordinator	1.0	12,000. 100%	12,000. 100%										
5	Transportation Aide	.50	5,500. 100%	5,500. 100%										
	TOTALS		$46,328	$46,328	$		$		$		$		$	

MCHRD 3/82   CONP PLN – 2221 – 001:1 N

HRD APPROVAL No.

MI – Staffing Worksheet

143

SCHEDULE III, SERVICE BUDGET WORKSHEET AND JUSTIFICATION NOTES

PSAL Programs, Inc. for   Page 1 of 1 pages

AGENCY NAME: Adult Day Care Center   FOR PERIOD: 10/1/83   TO: 9/30/84   PREPARED BY/DATE:

Budget Item	Budget	Budget	New Adult Day Care Program (20 - 50 clients) Agency Justification/Basis for Proposed Costs
PERSONNEL	$	$46,328.	See Schedule I
E.R.E.		7,843.	See Schedule II
PROF./O.S. SVCS.		2,400.	Janitorial
TRAVEL		6,960.	Participant: 1200 mi. mo x 12 mos. x 40¢ = $5,760 Staff: 500 mi. mo x 12 mos. x 20¢ = 1,200
SPACE		3,100.	Rent: $200 mo x 12 mos. = $2,400 Telephone: $58.33 mo. x 12 mos. = $700
EQUIPMENT		500.	2 tables @ $200 each, 5 chairs @ $20 each
MATERIALS/ SUPPLIES		10,831.	Food $1.78 meal x 20 participants x 252 days $8,971. Crafts $100 mo. x 12 mos. 1,200. Office Supplies $41.66 mo. x 12 mos. 500. Printing 60. Postage 500 stamps x 20¢ 100.
OPERATING SERVICES		590	Personnel Advertising 50. Insurance Liability. 540.
TOTAL DIRECT COSTS INDIRECT (11%)		78,552. 8,640	
TOTAL		$87,192	

MCHRD 3/82   COMP PLN - 2221 - 003:1 N   HRD APPROVAL NO.

M2 - Budget Worksheet

For Product Safety Concerns and Information please contact our EU
representative GPSR@taylorandfrancis.com
Taylor & Francis Verlag GmbH, Kaufingerstraße 24, 80331 München, Germany

www.ingramcontent.com/pod-product-compliance
Ingram Content Group UK Ltd.
Pitfield, Milton Keynes, MK11 3LW, UK
UKHW040926180425
457613UK00004B/40